Inadequate Care of the Elderly:
A Health Care Perspective
on Abuse and Neglect

Terry T. Fulmer, Ph.D., R.N., is an Associate Professor of Nursing at Boston College, Chestnut Hill, Massachusetts, and Associate Director of the Harvard Geriatric Education Center at Harvard Medical School in Boston, Massachusetts. She received her B.S. degree from Skidmore College and her M.S. and Ph.D. from Boston College. She has published numerous articles and chapters on the subject of elder abuse and gerontological nursing. She has received the Massachusetts Nurses Association award for nursing practice as well as the District V Nurses Association award for excellence in nursing education. She is Chairman of the Elder Abuse Assessment Team at the Beth Israel Hospital in Boston, where she is also on the staff of the Emergency Unit.

Terrence A. O'Malley, M.D., is engaged in the practice of internal medicine at the Massachusetts General Hospital, Boston, where he is the physician advisor to the Elder Care Committee and medical director of the Nursing Home Managed Care Program. Dr. O'Malley received his B.A. from Amherst College and his M.D. from Cornell University Medical College and completed his internship and residency in primary care internal medicine at MGH. He is an Instructor in Medicine at Harvard Medical School and is active in graduate and postgraduate medical education. He is on the professional advisory committees of several home care agencies, medical director of a local nursing home, and active in the care of a large number of homebound and institutionalized elderly persons. He has published extensively on the issues of abuse and neglect of the elderly.

INADEQUATE CARE
OF THE ELDERLY
A HEALTH CARE PERSPECTIVE
ON ABUSE AND NEGLECT

Terry T. Fulmer, Ph.D., R.N.
Terrence A. O'Malley, M.D.

SPRINGER PUBLISHING COMPANY
New York

Copyright © 1987 by Springer Publishing Company, Inc.

Springer Publishing Company, Inc.
536 Broadway
New York, NY 10012

87 88 89 90 91 / 5 4 3 2 1

Library of Congress Cataloging-in-Publication Data

Fulmer, Terry.
  Inadequate care of the elderly.

  Includes bibliographies and index.
  1. Long-term care of the sick. 2. Aged—Care.
3. Aged—Medical care. 4. Aged—Abuse of.
I. O'Malley, Terrence A. II. Title. [DNLM:
1. Elder Abuse. 2. Long Term Care—in old age.
WT 30 F973i]
RA997.F85   1987   362.1'0880565   87-9749
ISBN 0-8261-4770-4 (soft)

Printed in the United States of America

Contents

Introduction

This book is written for the health care professional responsible for elderly clients who are receiving inadequate care. This book is not a theoretical discussion of the causes of abuse and neglect, nor is it an exhaustive review of the literature. We present a practical perspective on abuse and neglect of the elderly that we hope will prove useful to the practitioner who must confront the ethical and logistical issues that make cases of abuse and neglect so difficult to manage.

This perspective starts with the contention that abuse and neglect of the elderly can best be thought of as part of a continuum of care rather than as separate entities. In this view, the provision of care to elderly persons can be judged to be either adequate or inadequate in amount and type. The presence of current care needs along with risk for further harm characterize the situation of elderly persons who are receiving inadequate care. There are many causes of inadequate care, but the effects on the elderly person are very similar whether it is caused by ignorance, disability, abuse, or neglect. Thus, the first task of the health care professional is to identify inadequate care.

Formulating the problem as "abuse" and "neglect" makes it impossible to include elderly persons who show signs of neglect of medical problems because they cannot afford care, do not have easy access to care, or are receiving care from well-meaning but inadequately trained caretakers. Without a broader definition, many elder persons who experience dangerously inadequate care would not receive assistance from a service system that is oriented only toward identifying cases of abuse and neglect perpetrated by caretakers, families, or institutions.

"Inadequate care" encompasses a wider group of elderly who are at risk for further harm, while including those who are the targets of intentional mistreatment. It also shifts the implied focus of intervention to the existence of inadequate care rather than to ascertaining its mechanisms and apportioning blame for its occurrence. In this way the needs of the elderly person are more clearly recognized and dealt with.

There are differences between what a practitioner must do to manage a case of inadequate care that results from willful interference by a caretaker and a case in which a similar degree of inadequate care results from the lack of a caretaker or a caretaker's ignorance of proper technique. One difference is the need to assess the possibility of separating the elderly person from the source of abuse versus providing better home care. In addition, in an abusive situation the practitioner must assess the need to engage the abuser in a therapeutic relationship. However, important as these issues are, the central concern of the practitioner is to identify and develop strategies to meet the care needs and ensure the safety of the elderly person.

We do, however, discuss abuse and neglect in this book as separate, distinct entities from inadequate care. We describe the physical signs that sometimes indicate the presence of abuse, and we discuss those situations that appear to place the elderly person at greater risk for abuse and neglect. We do this so that the practitioner can identify abuse when it clearly presents itself and can initiate the appropriate steps to separate the elderly person from the abusive situation if necessary. However, it is important to maintain the perspective of abuse as a subset of inadequate care.

The advantages of this approach are several. It is far easier to reach consensus on what constitutes adequate care than it is to define what constitutes abuse or neglect. This makes it easier for the service system to work in concert.

Those cases that do not meet the definition of abuse and neglect do not have to be ignored. They can still be given priority for services. There is little reason to have a separate system for dealing with abuse and neglect. Instead, one needs to have special capabilities within the existing system of social and protective services for dealing with cases in which the caretaker promotes or creates the inadequate care. With this outlook, restrictions on prioritization and case selection are removed, and these decisions can be made on the basis of need rather on statutory grounds.

The issue for the practitioner, then, is how to assure adequate care for the elderly person in the face of lack of services, active opposition by caretakers, or intentionally harmful activities by caretakers. This is not easy. Some cases that have been identified under the abuse and neglect reporting statutes are among the most difficult imaginable. However, by concentrating on the needs of the elderly person rather than on the actions of the caretaker, the practitioner will be in a better position to help improve the elderly person's situation.

Foreword

Inadequate care of the elderly? A confusing title at first glance—is this a handbook for treating older persons badly? An exposé of nursing home atrocities? A thin disguise for yet another health policy treatise on revamping Medicare? It is none of the above.

This volume represents a milestone in a rapidly evolving aspect of geriatrics, the assessment and correction of the mismatch between care provided and care needed. The concept of inadequate care goes well beyond the appropriate choice of antibiotics or proper surgical management of a fractured hip to deal broadly with unmet medical or social needs. This concept has developed from programs targeting elder abuse. In the late 1970s, elder abuse teams flourished. These interdisciplinary groups, charged with identification of cases, were hampered by the lack of a clear definition of abuse. In the setting of occasional sensational media coverage and the passage in many states of mandatory reporting requirements, early elder abuse teams sometimes become "search and destroy missions." I recall instances in which the label "abuser" was pinned on practitioners or institutions that were clearly more a part of the solution than the problem. Lengthy discussions resulted on who and what should be reported. What would be gained by punishing or trying to close a relatively well-run nursing home because of the actions of one of its employees in the midst of a disastrous shortage of nursing home beds? Would community elders be well served by reporting to the state the only practitioner in town willing to care for frail, poor, homebound, minority elders in the ghetto because one of his diabetic patients was inadequately managed?

It was clear from the beginning that while elder abuse exists and needs to be prevented it represents just the tip of a much larger iceberg of unmet needs. From its uncertain and sometimes awkward beginning the "Elder Abuse Movement" has matured remarkably. The focus has been expanded beyond abuse to include neglect, and largely through the efforts of Fulmer and O'Malley, the authors of this volume, this perspective has recently been broadened even further into inadequate care. The theme has changed from punishment of the perpetrator to identification of patients at risk and understanding and correcting the practices and conditions associated with unmet needs.

The insights, perspective, and strategies offered in this volume should be incorporated into the training and the practice of all health care providers dedicated to meeting the care needs of frail elders.

John W. Rowe, M.D.
Director
Harvard Geriatric Education Center
Boston, Massachusetts

1

Scope of the Problem and Causative Factors

The number of elderly people in America is increasing dramatically each year. Every day 1,000 people are added to the ranks of the over-65 population presently constituting 12 percent of our population. With advances in medical technology and pharmaceutical sophistication, we are noting a rapid growth in the segment of the population over 75 years of age, called the "old-old" or "frail elderly." Innovative medical advances such as pacemakers, renal dialysis procedures, and the many antibiotic therapies have brought about the phenomenon of "death control" (Rowe & Besdine, 1982).

We can project that, by the year 2020, 17 percent of the American population will be "elderly," that is, over 65 years of age. This population shift will place new and difficult demands on our society. Today, more than ever before, a middle-aged adult is likely to have one or both parents still living. The average life expectancy is now 70 years for males and 78 years for females. And when the post–World War II baby boom generation approaches the 65-year-old mark, we can expect an elderly majority.

As the elderly population increases, other significant changes are occurring. Traditionally, the female offspring has functioned as the care providers for aged parents, usually by bringing an aging parent into her home or arranging for living quarters in close proximity to her. Today, with approximately 50 percent of all married women in the labor force, it is less clear who the logical choice is for providing supportive care to elderly family members. In addition, modern advances in family planning will have left us with fewer adult children to act as caretakers for our elderly. The rising number of frail elderly persons, coupled with the decrease in numbers of potential family caretakers, may impact on the prevalence of elder abuse in the future. Housing trends and trends in the availability of community-based services to replace those traditionally provided by other family members will also have an impact on the prevalence of abuse and neglect. It is likely that the problem of inadequate care will grow.

SCOPE OF THE PROBLEM

What do we know about the scope of the problems of abuse and neglect? Six congressional hearings and a national study on elder abuse were conducted by the House Select Committee on Aging, which produced a report entitled *Elder Abuse: An Examination of a Hidden Problem* (U.S. House of Representatives, 1981). An overview of findings of that report have been summarized by Oakar and Miller (1983, pp. 431–432)[1].

1. Elder abuse is a full-scale national problem which exists with a frequency and rate only slightly less than that of child abuse.
2. An estimated 4% of the nation's elderly, one million older Americans, are victims of some sort of abuse, from moderate to severe, each year.
3. While one out of three cases of child abuse is reported, only one out of six cases of elder abuse comes to the attention of the authorities.

[1]Reproduced with permission from *Abuse and Maltreatment of the Elderly, Causes and Interventions*, by Jordan I. Kosberg. © 1983 by PSG Publishing Company, Inc., Littleton, Massachusetts.

4. The victims are likely to be very old—75 or older. Women are more often abused than men. The victims are usually in a position of dependency; i.e., they rely on others, often the persons who abuse them, for their care and protection.
5. The probable abuser will undoubtedly be experiencing great stress. Alcoholism, drug addiction, marital problems, and long-term financial difficulties are often factors in abuse of older persons.
6. The most likely abuser is the son of the victim (21% of cases) followed by the daughter (17% of cases). The third most frequent abuser is the spouse who acts in a caregiver role, with the male spouse more likely to be the abuser than the female spouse.
7. Older persons are less likely to report abuse, because they are ashamed, do not wish to bring trouble to the family, are afraid of reprisals, or do not have the physical ability to register complaints.

Current estimates suggest that between 0.5 and 1.4 million American elders are victims of abuse, neglect, exploitation, or abandonment each year. While most experts believe it occurs with approximately the same frequency as child abuse, which is the focus of well-organized legal and social welfare programs, elderly abuse has received little attention and accounts for only 7 percent of all preventive services provided to U.S. citizens (U.S. Senate and House, 1980).

The terms *abuse* and *neglect of the elderly* are used to describe situations in which individuals over the age of 65 experience battering, verbal abuse, exploitation, denial of rights, forced confinement, neglected medical needs, or other types of personal harm, usually at the hands of someone responsible for assisting them in their activities of daily living (O'Malley, Everitt, O'Malley, & Campion, 1983). Several studies have documented the range of seriousness of this form of violence. Burns, oversedation, malnutrition, dehydration, decubiti, inappropriate medication dosages, fractures, concussions, freezing, and sexual abuse have all been reported (O'Malley, Segars, Perez, Mitchell, & Knuepel, et al., 1979).

In the studies conducted to date, the most common profile

of the abused older person is of a female over 75 years of age who is frail and multiply dependent and usually presents with health care needs concerning hygiene, nutrition, safety, toileting, and orientation. In a summary paper of these research studies (O'Rourke, 1981), a profile of the abused victim is outlined for each of the studies discussed (see Table 1-1).

Since females have a longer life expectancy than males, it is not surprising that they are more frequently cited as elder abuse victims. There has been much debate regarding the validity of the abuse-victim profiles listed in Table 1-1. A major and central issue is the fact that each study used a different definition. Small samples and various research approaches also detract from the studies' ability to predict potential or actual victims. Callahan (1981) reminds us that, to date, "abuse, like beauty, is in the eye of the beholder" (p. 2). However, he is willing to accept some of the data from these studies, those indicating that victims of abuse usually are very old, functionally impaired, living with others, and abused by a relative.

Since those early studies, researchers have used different approaches to avoid such methodological difficulties. One such method has been to confine research to physical abuse only (Pillemer, 1985). Another has been to set up multiple

TABLE 1-1 Profiles of Abuse Victims as Summarized by O'Rourke (1981)

Massachusetts (1979)	Maryland (1979)	Ohio (1979)
Old-old	Old-old	No age given
Female	Female	Severely impaired
Physically & mentally impaired	Protestant	Female
Living with others	Middle class	Widow
Not isolated	Living with relatives	White
	Moderately or severely mentally or physically impaired	Living with relatives

testing sites which vary geographically (Wolf, Godkin, & Pillemer, 1984). These later descriptions of the abused elderly are similar to the earlier studies.

The same studies that have put forth a profile of the abuse victim have offered an abuser profile as well, with similar methodological problems. A profile of elder abusers usually depicts them as being under some situational stress such as the loss of employment or divorce. They may be substance abusers, coping with the effects of alcoholism or drug addiction, or they may have a known psychiatric history. The issue of stress predominates the characterization, and usually some crisis in their lives has preceded the alleged abuse event. To date, it is not clear whether a relative or nonrelative is more likely to be an abuser, but some studies (Block & Sinnott, 1979) indicate that family members are more likely to be abusers.

FACTORS INVOLVED IN ELDER ABUSE

Douglass, Hickey, and Noele (1980) propose the following hypotheses of factors related to abuse, based on the current theories:

1. Dependence incurred in old age increases the risk of abuse or neglect.
2. A child who is abused or who witnesses abuse grows up to be an abusive adult.
3. Life crises, in either the abused or the abuser, may trigger abusive behavior.
4. Environmental factors play a major force in bringing about neglectful or abusive behavior.

To date, there are five major groups of theories of causation for elder abuse. In an individual case it is extremely difficult to separate one theory from another because, so often, the complex nature of the situation encompasses components of several theories. However, for the purpose of providing a theoretical background, each of these five will be presented separately. A more comprehensive discussion of theories of causation for elder abuse appears elsewhere (Pillemer & Wolf, 1986).

Impairment of the Older Person

The impairment theories advance the idea that an elderly person who has a severe physical or mental impairment is most likely to be abused (Block & Sinnott, 1979). We must be careful here to note that being impaired does not mean that the victims have *caused* their abuse. Rather, because of their impairment, they are likely to be dependent and are therefore highly *vulnerable* to abuse and neglect. While only 5 percent of the nation's elderly are in long-term care institutions, 45 percent of the population over 62 years of age experiences some limitation of activity due to chronic conditions (USDHEW, 1979); thus, people have an increasing proportion of dependency needs as they advance in age.

The following case illustrates an example that falls into this category.

A working mother of two teenage children brought her own mother to the emergency room and stated that she couldn't do it anymore. On physical examination, the 82-year-old mother was found to have a fractured hip and a deep decubitus ulcer on her sacrum. The social history revealed that the daughter left her mother at home alone during the day because she could not afford home health aide services. As she found her mother to be more of a burden, she admitted to shoving her and causing her to fall, because "she was always in the way." The fall had occurred one week prior to the emergency unit visit. Since that time, the mother had been immobile and lying on her back, which was the presumed cause of her decubitus. The tearful daughter had no idea that her mother's hip was broken.

Psychopathology of the Abuser

The psychopathology theories focus on the abuser and contend that abusers have personality traits or character disorders that cause them to be abusive. The following case history is illustrative.

An elderly woman presented in the emergency unit with an admitting diagnosis of pneumonia. Upon physical examination, it was noted that she had multiple facial bruises and upper-arm contusions. She was extremely withdrawn and asked the nurses "not to hit her." A social history revealed that her two sons, with whom she lived, had both been diagnosed as psychotic and were currently on medications for their mental problems. Paradoxically, they identified themselves as extremely devoted to their mother and had initiated the medical treatment for her pneumonia symptoms. Despite the physical abuse she was subject to, the mother chose her home setting with her sons as preferable to long-term care placement or removal of the sons from her home.

The term *non-normal caregiver* (Lau & Kosberg, 1979) has also been applied to mentally retarded offspring or alcoholic offspring who may not have the decision-making capacity to make appropriate judgments regarding the needs of their elderly parents. Drug and alcohol dependency may result in financial exploitation, intimidation, and battering.

Transgenerational Violence

The theories of transgenerational violence hold that violence is a learned, normative behavior pattern in some families. As a child is growing up, he observes violence as an accepted reaction to stress and internalizes it as a behavior. This leads to a cyclical familial pattern in which the abused child becomes an abuser of his or her parents, spouse, or children. The following case illustrates this theory.

As a youth, Mr. S was terribly afraid of his father, an alcoholic who was frequently absent from the home but who, when he did return, often beat the children and his wife in angry outbursts of temper. Mr. S recalls hating him. As his father's health deteriorated from his alcoholism, he became debilitated and spent most of his time in the home. Mr. S recalls "slugging him whenever he lipped-off," in retaliation for his father's previous abusiveness.

Stressed Caretaker

The stressed caretaker theories emphasize the relationship between stress and its translation into abuse or neglect. It is not important whether the stress results from sources external to the family or from the demands of caring for a dependent elderly parent. Some caregivers report somatic and psychosomatic complaints such as headaches, insomnia, depression, and anxiety because of their perceived stress. Block and Sinnott (1979) discuss how adult children exhibit frustration and resentment toward their elders in the family context where the dependency of the oldest family member is an unexpected burden of extended duration. This theory contends that, as internal stresses mount, abuse is likely to result. The following case is an example of this theory.

Upon her father's unexpected death, Mrs. R took her mother home to live with her. Her mother was 75 years old and had been in poor health for some time, but her father had always been able to care for her. About a month after her mother's arrival, Mrs. R sought medical treatment for unrelieved migraine headaches. As the headaches continued she became increasingly short with her mother and began giving her extra sleeping medications to "keep her out of her hair." The physician treating Mrs. R's migraine headaches was finally able to elicit the story about the extra medications and intervene with support services before any major crisis occurred.

External stresses include changes in income, employment status, and marital status, all of which may have an impact on the incidence of abuse. O'Malley (1979) reports that the abuser is likely to be experiencing some form of external stress at the time of abuse. Douglass et al. (1980) suggest that life crises such as the loss of a job, divorce, a change in residence, or decrease in income could impact family dynamics in a negative direction, triggering abuse. The following is one such case.

> Mr. and Mrs. M had two young children, and Mrs. M's mother had lived with them for four years without incident. When Mr. M lost his job, he became increasingly resentful of the medical expenses incurred by his mother-in-law and began to neglect her needs. The older woman's health declined significantly from the lack of medical attention. A hospital admission was finally warranted for congestive heart failure, and nursing home placement followed.

Exchange Theory

An important new contribution to the understanding of abuse and neglect is the so-called "exchange theory" proposed by Pillemer (1984). This model looks at the relationship between the abusive person and the abused victim and postulates that abuse will occur as long as the abuser gains from it. When the exchange becomes unfavorable (due to threat of sanctions, fear, lack of monetary return, guilt), then the abuser is likely to cease. This may help explain why the mere presence of any outsider in the home of an abuse victim may stop abuse by raising the possibility of sanctions. This is true even when no tangible benefit (such as help with caretaking) is provided. Finally, the social isolation theory proposes that since violence is an unacceptable behavior in our society, violent activity is intentionally hidden. This theory postulates that the introduction of others into a family situation results in a decrease in violent behavior due to a "watch dog" effect. Since research has documented that physically abused elders are more socially isolated than non-abused elders (Pillemer, 1984), it is important to consider the benefits that may result from placing an additional person in the home of an elder.

SUMMARY

Although research into the scope and causes of abuse and neglect are still in the preliminary stages, the studies cited here have demonstrated that abuse and neglect is a potentially significant problem for all elderly persons regardless of socioeconomic status. The aging of society makes it likely that it will grow in importance over the next several decades. Although the theories advance to explain abuse and neglect are helpful, intervention strategies are being developed empirically by trial and error, and we are still searching for theoretical justification for their effectiveness.

At this point in the evolution of our understanding and study of the problems of abuse and neglect, we are facing two conflicting needs. The first is to better define the theoretical underpinnings of the causes of abuse and neglect, and the other is to perfect strategies for intervention and prevention. The basis of this difficulty rests on our current definitions of abuse and neglect. This issue is discussed further in the following chapter.

REFERENCES

Block, M., & Sinnott, J. (Eds.) (1979). *The Battered Elder Syndrome: An Exploratory Study.* College Park, MD: University of Maryland, Center on Aging.

Callahan, J. J. (1981, March 23–25, April 1–3). *Elder Abuse Programming— Will It Help the Elderly?* Paper presented at the National Conference on the Abuse of Older Persons. Boston and San Francisco.

Douglass, R. L., Hickey, T., & Noele, C. (1980). *A Study of Maltreatment of the Elderly and Other Vulnerable Adults.* Ann Arbor, MI: University of Michigan, Institute of Gerontology.

Lau, E., & Kosberg, J. I. (1979). Abuse of the Elderly by Informal Care Providers. *Aging, 229,* 5–10.

Oakar, M. R., & Miller, C. A. (1983). Federal Legislation to Protect the Elderly. In J. I. Kosberg (Ed.), *Abuse and Maltreatment of the Elderly: Causes and Interventions* (pp. 422–435). Littleton, MA: John Wright/ PSG, Inc.

O'Malley, T. A., Everitt, D. C., O'Malley, H. C., & Campion, E. W. (1983, June). Identifying and Preventing Family-Mediated Abuse and Neglect of Elderly Persons. *Annals of Internal Medicine, 98*(6), 998–1005.

O'Malley, H. C., Segars, H., Perez, R., Mitchell, V., & Knuepel, G. M., et al. (1979). *Elder Abuse in Massachusetts: A Survey of Professionals and Paraprofessionals.* Boston: Legal Research and Services for the Elderly.

O'Rourke, M. (1981, March 23–25, April 1–3). *Elder Abuse—The State of the Art.* Paper prepared for the National Conference on the Abuse of Older Persons. Boston and San Francisco.

Pillemer, C. N., & Wolf, R. (Eds.). (1986). *Elder abuse: Conflict in the family.* Dover, MA: Auburn House.

Pillemer, K. (1984, December). *The Dangers of Dependency: New Findings on Domestic Violence against the Elderly.* Unpublished paper. Durham, NH: University of New Hampshire, Family Violence Research Program.

Pillemer, K. (1985). Social Isolation and Elder Abuse. *Response, 8*(4), 2–4.

Rowe, J. W., & Besdine, R. W. (1982). *Health and Disease in Old Age.* Boston: Little, Brown.

U.S. Department of Health Education and Welfare, Public Health Service. (1979). *The National Nursing Home Survey: 1977 Summary for the United States.* DHEW Publication No. (PHS) 79-1974. Washington, DC: U.S. Government Printing Office.

U.S. House of Representatives, Select Committee on Aging. (1981). *Elder abuse: An examination of a hidden problem.* (Comm. Pub. No. 97-277). Washington, DC: U.S. Government Printing Office.

U.S. Senate and U.S. House of Representatives. (1980, June 11). Joint Hearing before the Special Committee on Aging, U.S. Senate and the Select Committee on Aging, U.S. House of Representatives, Ninety-sixth Congress.

Wolf, R., Godkin, M., & Pillemer, K. (1984). *Elder Abuse and Neglect: Final Report from Three Model Projects.* Worcester, MA: University of Massachusetts, Center on Aging.

2

The Difficulty of Defining Abuse and Neglect

There are no universally accepted definitions of abuse and neglect of the elderly. In part this is due to significant differences that exist in the standards that are applied by the various ethnic and religious subgroups in our population to behavior between parents, children, and spouses. Behavior that is accepted by one group as appropriate for dealing with discipline or differences of opinion within the family may be labeled "family violence" by another group. Raising one's voice, shouting insults, depriving someone of food or privileges, forcing confinement to a separate room, striking with the hand, striking with a belt or other instrument, battering, or inflicting serious injury are part of the spectrum of behavior used to enforce discipline or resolve disputes within families.

As one moves toward the more physical and injurious behaviors there are fewer families in which such behaviors are common or accepted. However, in 70 percent of families surveyed in a recent comprehensive study of family violence (Straus, Gelles, & Steinmetz, 1980), the right to inflict serious injury was felt to be a parental prerogative.

The issue of acceptable limits on parental behavior has been extensively discussed in the child abuse literature, and behavior that endangers the physical or mental health of the child is considered to be unacceptable and subject to action by society. In the case of the vulnerable and dependent child, society has assumed the responsibility for defining acceptable behavior and acting on the child's behalf to protect him from abuse by his parents. In most statutes, this responsibility extends to assuring that the child's needs for food, shelter, clothing, and medical care are also met, thereby permitting the state to intervene in instances of neglect of basic needs as well as for episodes of physical abuse. Abandonment is the most extreme form of neglect and is recognized under most of the child abuse statutes.

Similar issues exist in the area of abuse and neglect of the elderly. Frail, vulnerable elders who are dependent on others to meet their requirements for care are in a position analogous to that of children. However, there has not been an extensive discussion on the limits of acceptable behavior of children toward their aging parents. Although the comparison of elder abuse and child abuse may help society focus on acceptable standards of behavior within families, this comparison doesn't capture the full extent of the issues created by abuse and neglect of the elderly.

The natural history of chronic and acute illness in the elderly may mask the presence of abuse or neglect because it is difficult to determine whether the elderly person's worsening physical condition is due to the natural progression of illness or to omissions or active interventions on the part of a caretaker. This is usually not a problem in child abuse, where developmental norms are well established and where any deviations from the expected continued growth and development of the child are viewed with concern. But in the elderly there are no norms of aging with which to compare the suspected case of abuse or neglect. The confusion over whether abuse or neglect has occurred compounds the difficulty of establishing the role of inappropriate caretaker behaviors in causing abuse or neglect, thereby making any definition difficult to apply.

To illustrate, while it is known that as a part of the normal aging process there is, for example, increased capillary fragility, osteoporosis, decreased vital capacity, and decreased visual acuity, it is not known what a "normal" or "acceptable" fracture or bruise looks like compared with an injury resulting from abuse of an elderly person. Figure 2–1 is a schematic depiction of the possible cumulative effects of age plus disease plus neglect.

The problem presented by Figure 2–1 is that there is no way to "weight" each of these factors. Are the changes that come with age more clinically notable than the changes that result from neglect? Are neglect indicators more obvious than symptoms of disease? To date, no one has been able to answer these questions. It is therefore difficult to establish a definition of abuse and neglect on the basis of physical signs.

Clinical examples give another perspective on this issue, as illustrated in Table 2–1. Each example is meant to illustrate the complexity of determining whether abnormal findings are age related, disease related, or the result of neglect. Elders over 65 years of age have an average of 3.5 chronic health problems each (Rowe & Besdine, 1982). It is ex-

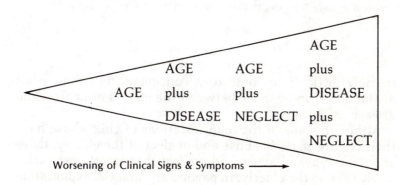

Worsening of Clinical Signs & Symptoms ⟶

FIGURE 2–1 Possible cumulative effects of age, disease, and neglect

Source: Fulmer, T. & Ashley, J. 1986. Neglect: What Part of Abuse? *Pride Institute Journal of Long Term Home Health Care*, 5(4), p. 21. Reprinted with permission.

TABLE 2-1 Two Examples of Indicators of Neglect, with Possible Causes

Indicator of Neglect	Possible Causes			
	Age	Age plus Disease	Age plus Neglect	Age plus Disease plus Neglect
Fracture	Osteoporosis	Osteoporosis plus stress fracture	Osteoporosis plus inadequate assistance with ambulation	Osteoporosis plus stress fracture due to inadequate assistance with ambulation
Poor hygiene	Decreased visual acuity	Decreased visual acuity plus rheumatoid arthritis	Decreased visual acuity plus inadequate self-washing leading to poor hygiene	Decreased visual acuity plus rheumatoid arthritis (pain) leading to inadequate self-washing & resultant poor hygiene

Adapted from: Fulmer, T. & Ashley, J. 1986, Neglect: What Part of Abuse? *Pride Institute Journal of Long Term Health Care, 5*(4), p. 21. Used with permission.

tremely difficult to come to a consensus regarding what distinctions can be made between the effects of neglect and disease in old age.

Although some of the manifestations of child abuse have their counterparts in abuse and neglect of the elderly, there are some types of abuse and neglect that are almost exclusively seen in the elderly. In particular, financial exploitation is commonly seen with the elderly. The reason for this is that the elderly frequently have assets such as pensions, savings, or property. Financial vulnerability is coupled with physical vulnerability in abuse of the elderly. The management of assets within the family may or may not involve the participation of the elderly person; and the possibility of exploitation exists.

In cases of child abuse, society imposes its definition on the family and can enforce its decisions by intervening in situations that threaten the well-being of the child. Society's options are more limited in the case of abuse or neglect of an adult. The elderly person is the only one who can determine the limits of behavior that are acceptable to him or her and give permission for intervention. Although society can develop general descriptions of behaviors that it considers unacceptable, only the elderly person can decide if those definitions apply in his or her individual case. In a sense, the elderly person can render a definition of abuse or neglect meaningless. If nothing can be done to ameliorate a situation because the elderly person refuses to acknowledge the existence of abuse or neglect, then there is little to be gained by identifying cases in this manner. This imposes a very practical limit on the utility of definitions of abuse and neglect. Any definitions must facilitate the elderly person's acceptance of intervention; otherwise, they will be counterproductive.

Despite these difficulties, some definitions of abuse and neglect have been proposed. Table 2-2 lists examples of the various definitions which have been used by researchers, legislators, and service professionals. This list is by no means comprehensive, but it is meant to illustrate the variations and discrepancies in such definitions to date. A complete review of definitions has been compiled by Johnson (1986) which breaks out each definition by behavioral manifestations.

We have found that none of these definitions is adequate for the purpose of defining cases that require sociomedical (rather than legal) intervention. Most are too restrictive and omit cases that could benefit from intervention, even though there is no abuse or neglect according to the definition. Some restrict their definitions to a particular category of elderly persons, such as those who live at home with family, or those who live in institutions. Others restrict

TABLE 2-2 Definitions of Elder Abuse

Source	Definition
O'Malley, Segars, & Perez (1979), adapted from Connecticut Department of Aging	*Abuse*: The willful infliction of physical pain, injury, or debilitating mental anguish; unreasonable confinement; or deprivation by a caretaker of services which are necessary to maintain mental and physical health.
Block & Sinnott (1979)	1. *Physical abuse*: malnutrition; injuries, e.g., bruises, welts, sprains, dislocations, abrasions, or lacerations. 2. *Psychological abuse*: verbal assault, threat, fear, isolation. 3. *Material abuse*: theft, misuse of money or property. 4. *Medical abuse*: withholding of medications or aids required.
Douglass, Hickey, & Noele (1980)	1. *Passive neglect*: being ignored, left alone, isolated, forgotten. 2. *Active neglect*: withholding of companionship, medicine, food, exercise, assistance to bathroom. 3. *Verbal or emotional abuse*: name-calling, insults, treating as a child, frightening humiliation, intimidation, threats. 4. *Physical abuse*: being hit, slapped, bruised, sexually molested, cut, burned, physically restrained.
Lau & Kosberg (1979)	1. *Physical abuse*: direct beatings; withholding personal care, food, medical care; lack of supervision. 2. *Psychological abuse*: verbal assaults, threats, provoking fear, isolation. 3. *Material abuse*: monetary or material theft or misuse. 4. *Violation of rights*: being forced out of one's dwelling or forced into another setting.
Wolf & Pillemer (1984)	1. *Physical abuse*: the infliction of physical pain or injury, physical coercion (confinement against one's will), e.g., slapped, bruised, sexually molested, cut, burned, physically restrained.

TABLE 2-2 (Continued)

Source	Definition
	2. *Psychological abuse*: the infliction of mental anguish, e.g., called names, treated as child, frightened, humiliated, intimidated, threatened, isolated. 3. *Material abuse*: the illegal or improper exploitation and/or use of funds or other resources. 4. *Active neglect*: refusal or failure to fulfill a caretaking obligation, including a conscious and intentional attempt to inflict physical or emotional stress on the elder; e.g., deliberate abandonment or deliberate denial of food or health-related services. 5. *Passive neglect*: refusal or failure to fulfill a caretaking obligation, excluding a conscious and intentional attempt to inflict physical or emotional distress on the elder; e.g., abandonment, nonprovision of food or health-related services because of inadequate knowledge, laziness, infirmity, or disrupting the value of prescribed services.
O'Malley, Everitt, O'Malley, & Campion (1984)	1. *Neglect*: failure of a caretaker to intervene to resolve a significant need despite awareness of available resources. 2. *Abuse*: active intervention by a caretaker such that unmet needs are created or sustained with resultant physical, psychological, or financial injury.

cases to those that have resulted from some demonstrable behavior on the part of the "abuser" such as the "acts" of abuse, neglect, abandonment, or exploitation.

Some of these definitions include the terms *self-neglect*, *active neglect*, and *passive neglect*, which have been advanced to describe various processes by which inadequate care can result. In self-neglect the individual is responsible for the results of his own inaction, whether that is due to ignorance, disinclination to act, or unwillingness or inability to identify a problem. This category is only helpful if one is trying to separate elderly persons whose inadequate care is the result of their own action or inaction from those elderly persons whose inadequate care is the result of someone else's action or inaction.

This is an important distinction for protective service systems to make if they are mandated to intervene only in cases of neglect that result from the actions or inactions of a responsible third party. In the latter context, *active neglect* is used to describe behavior by a responsible party that is directed toward intentionally impeding necessary intervention designed to resolve an unmet need. *Passive neglect* describes situations in which a responsible party takes no measures to intervene, despite knowledge of an unmet need.

Distinctions between types of neglect, however, have very little utility for the physician, nurse, or social worker, except perhaps when developing an intervention strategy. Even then, their value is limited because it is difficult to characterize the actions of the inadequate caretaker as simply "active" or "passive."

There is no apparent logic behind the pattern of choices of elder abuse or neglect definitions by various states. Thobaben and Anderson (1985), in their review of state reporting laws, point out the variation among the definitions that are currently in use across the country. Differences in what is covered under mandatory reporting laws are also described. At this time, it has not been determined how well the various definitions have worked in practice, so there are no objective results with which to compare definitions. The irreconcilable problem with these definitions is that they are too narrow to encompass fully the problems confronted by the health care professional. As such, they are too restrictive to be useful and instead produce as many difficulties as they seek to resolve.

This is due mostly to the fact that these definitions evolved from a research perspective rather than a patient-care perspective. The researcher must try to develop homogeneous groups and thereby eliminate as many variables as possible. Otherwise, interpretation of experimental results is impossible because of confounding variables. The practitioner's goals are very different and are the ones that we are pursuing in this book. The practitioner seeks to identify cases of abuse and neglect solely in order to resolve them because they represent elderly persons who are receiving inadequate care.

These two approaches are incompatible and cannot be reconciled. It is important to realize this and proceed with designing intervention systems that are service oriented rather than research oriented. Many of the difficulties faced by the practitioner who attempts to manage cases using definitions in many of the current abuse reporting laws result from the inclusion of definitions that evolved from a research perspective rather than a service perspective. While both approaches are valid for their respective tasks, they cannot be used interchangeably.

How can the definition be changed to encompass the problem? All cases of abuse and neglect can be thought of as inadequate care, defined as the presence of unmet needs for personal care (see Figure 2–2). These needs include the basic requirements of food, shelter, and clothing as well as the needs for supportive relationships, freedom from harassment or threats or violence, and the opportunity to define an acceptable lifestyle. Other needs may include the requirement for assistance in the activities of daily living such as toileting, ambulating, dressing, eating, and managing medications and finances. One advantage of this construct is that abuse and neglect can be given a qualitative dimension (i.e., the type of unmet need) as well as a quantitative dimension (i.e., the extent or significance of the need), as can other "types" of inadequate care.

For the purpose of this book, as well as our own practice, we define elder abuse as "actions of a caretaker that create unmet needs for the elderly person," such as for food, shelter, supportive relationships, or medical care. We define

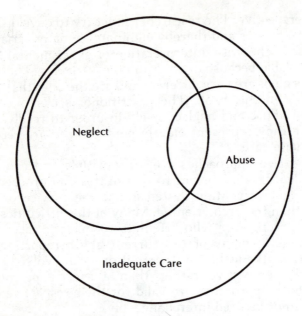

FIGURE 2-2 The universe of inadequate care.

neglect as "the failure of an individual responsible for caretaking to respond adequately to established needs for care."
In some cases, care needs result from the natural progression of disease or disability; in other cases they result from
the actions of someone other than the elderly person. The
concept of inadequate care can also be applied to situations
in which the only care need is for protection from threats or
violence directed at an elderly person who otherwise functions totally independently of others.

There are significant advantages to defining cases of
abuse and neglect as "inadequate care." It is easier to reach a
consensus on what constitutes adequate and inadequate
care than it is to agree upon what is acceptable and unacceptable behavior within families or among professionals. It is
easier to operationalize definitions of inadequate care because it is easier to identify. There is much less reluctance

on the part of health care professionals to identify inadequate care than there is to evoke the label of abuse or neglect.

Since inadequate care can exist without being caused by abuse or neglect, and since it is no less important to resolve inadequate care due to ignorance or lack of access to services than it is to resolve inadequate care that results from abuse or neglect, this definition more closely approximates what the health care professional actually faces. It can be applied to all elderly persons without regard to their living arrangements. It can be used for elderly persons who live alone and are unable to meet their own care needs (so called "self-neglect"), for those who are dependent on family members at home, for elders who are dependent on professional caretakers at home or in institutions, and for those who live independently but need protective services to defend themselves from assaults or exploitation.

This emphasis on the condition of the individual helps to focus interventions on the care needs of all elderly persons. We are able to respond to cases of abuse and neglect with only minor modifications in the approach that we use with any other inadequately cared for elder. In subsequent chapters we will describe this approach in detail and discuss techniques for dealing with the most troublesome aspects of case management.

Theories of abuse are important background for improving actual clinical assessment and postulating the causal relationships that result in inadequate care. In Chapter 9, the relationship between these theoretical models for inadequate care and the environment of the elder will be discussed.

REFERENCES

Block, M., & Sinnott, J. (Eds.). (1979). *The Battered Elder Syndrome: An Exploratory Study.* College Park, MD: University of Maryland, Center on Aging.

Douglass, R. L., Hickey, T., & Noele, C. (1980). *A Study of Maltreatment of the Elderly and Other Vulnerable Adults.* Ann Arbor, MI: University of Michigan, Institute of Gerontology.

Johnson, T. (1986). Critical Issues in the Definition of Elder Mistreatment. In Pillemer, C. A. & Wolf, R. S. (Eds.), *Elder Abuse: Conflict in the Family.* Dover, MA: Auburn House Publishing Company, pp. 167–270.

Lau, E., & Kosberg, J. I. (1979). Abuse of the Elderly by Informal Care Providers. *Aging, 229*(10), 5.

Oakar, M. R., & Miller, C. A. (1983). Federal Legislation to Protect the Elderly. In J. I. Kosberg (Ed.), *Abuse and Maltreatment of the Elderly: Causes and Interventions* (pp. 422–435). Littleton, MA: John Wright/PSG, Inc.

O'Malley, H. C., Segars, H. D., & Perez, R. (1979). *Elder Abuse in Massachusetts: A Survey of Professionals and Paraprofessionals.* Boston: Legal Research and Services for the Elderly.

O'Malley, T. A., Everitt, D. C., O'Malley, H. C., & Campion, E. W. (1983). Identifying and Preventing Family-Mediated Abuse and Neglect of Elderly Persons. *Annals of Internal Medicine, 98*(6, Pt. 1), 998–1005.

Rowe, J. W., & Besdine, R. W. (Eds.). (1982). *Health and Disease in Old Age.* Boston, MA: Little, Brown.

Straus, M. A., Gelles, R. J., & Steinmetz, S. K. (1980). *Behind Closed Doors.* Garden City, NY: Anchor Books.

Thobaben, M., & Anderson, L. (1985). Reporting Elder Abuse: It's the Law. *American Journal of Nursing, 85*(4), 371–374.

3

Identifying Abuse, Neglect, and Inadequate Care

It is important to identify inadequate care correctly because of the probability that it will continue and lead to further harm unless appropriate intervention is made. The need to intervene is not affected by the mechanism that caused the inadequate care or by the living arrangement of the elderly person. There is justification for action when the elderly person receives inadequate care because he or she lives alone and has no access to adequate services; lives with a family member and is battered, exploited, or neglected; or lives in an institution that provides substandard care.

MANIFESTATIONS OF INADEQUATE CARE

Inadequate care results from the presence of unmet needs for services or assistance which threaten the physical and psychological well-being of the individual. Most elderly persons who are receiving inadequate care present to the medical and nursing professions with manifestations that are predictable on the basis of their functional limitations and medical problems. The most common presentations involve combinations of poor hygiene, malnutrition, unmanaged medical problems, frequent falls, and confusion. Less frequently, legal or social services or the police are involved initially because of failure to meet financial obligations or because of abnormal behavior. The manifestations of "self-abuse and neglect" are primarily those of neglected medical problems, poor hygiene, malnutrition, and signs of deliberate self-injury. In caretaker-mediated abuse or neglect, as seen at home or in institutions, signs of battering, deliberate injury, pharmacological restraint through oversedation, and psychological manifestations of mistreatment may also be present.

Table 3–1 lists many of the manifestations of inadequate care, which, of course, includes those that result from abuse and neglect. The presence of these findings does not establish the diagnosis of neglect, since these same findings can result from the natural progression of some chronic illnesses. Despite this limitation, these signs suggest the presence of inadequate care.

Even though one may recognize inadequate care on the basis of these signs, one cannot identify the cause of the inadequate care. One cannot tell which elderly persons, solely on the basis of their presentation, have care needs that were known but not met by a responsible party and those whose care needs were known only to themselves. Nor, with a few exceptions, can one determine whether a particular manifestation of trauma is an expected consequence of an unmet care need or is the result of an intentionally inflicted injury by the individual or by another. All that can be concluded by the health care professional is that inadequate care is present and poses a potential risk to the well-being of the elderly person.

It may not be apparent why signs of trauma should be considered manifestations of inadequate care, since they imply active injury. Trauma can occur, however, as the result of accidental injury in situations in which there is lack of supervision, impaired cognition, or difficulty with ambulation. Injuries also occur in situations in which the care is totally adequate and there are no unmet needs for care. These signs of trauma are included to remind the health

TABLE 3-1 Manifestations of Inadequate Care

Abrasions	Dehydration
Lacerations	Malnutrition
Contusions	Inappropriate clothing
Burns	Poor hygiene
Freezing	Oversedation
Depression	Over- or under-medication
Fractures	Untreated medical problems
Sprains	Behavior that endangers the client or others
Dislocations	Failure to meet legal obligations
Decubiti	

care professional to assess not only the severity of the injury but also its mechanism and context in which it occurred, in order to identify causative factors that are correctable.

Abused elderly persons constitute another subset of elders receiving inadequate care. We define abuse here as the creation of care needs, and we expand care needs to include the need for protective services. As in child abuse, specific injuries such as bruises in the shape of hangers or buckles, or cigarette burns on the buttocks, back, or upper arms strongly suggest physical abuse (Rathbone-McCuan & Voyles, 1982). However, the manifestations of abuse and neglect in the elderly are usually more subtle. Rather than direct injuries, they are more frequently the signs of inadequately managed medical problems such as poorly controlled congestive heart failure or malnutrition. Although inadequate care can usually be diagnosed on the basis of an evaluation of the patient, the contribution of a caretaker or alleged abuser to the resulting injuries is never clear except in the most flagrant instances of battering. The physical manifestations of abuse can include all of those listed in Table 3-1. In addition, however, there are manifestations of abuse that are not shared with neglect. These are listed in Table 3-2.

In addition to observing these manifestations, health care professionals may also become aware of abuse on the basis

TABLE 3-2 Physical Indicators of Abuse Not Shared with Neglect

Unexplained bruises and welts:
  Face, lips, mouth
  Torso, back, buttocks, thighs
  In various stages of healing
  Clustered, forming regular patterns
  Reflecting shape of article used to inflict (electric cord, belt buckle)
  On several different surface areas
  Regularly appear after absence, weekend, or vacation
Unexplained burns:
  Cigar, cigarette burns, especially on soles, palms, back, or buttocks
  Immersion burns (sock-like on feet, glove-like on hands, doughnut-
    shaped on buttocks or genitalia)
  Patterned like electric burner, iron, etc.
  Rope burns on arms, legs, neck, or torso
Unexplained fractures:
  To skull, nose, facial structure
  In various stages of healing
  Multiple or spiral fractures
Unexplained lacerations or abrasions:
  To mouth, lips, gums, eyes
  To external genitalia
Sexual abuse:
  Difficulty in walking or sitting
  Torn, stained, or bloody underclothing
  Pain or itching in genital area
  Bruises or bleeding in external genitalia or in vaginal or anal areas
  Venereal disease

Source: Adapted from U.S. Department of Health, Education and Welfare, *Physical and Behavioral Indicators of Child Abuse and Neglect, Training in the Prevention and Treatment of Child Abuse and Neglect.* USDHEW Pub. No. (OHDS) 79-3021. 1979, pp. 47–48.

of the elderly person's behavior at the time of the interview. Reports of abuse by the elderly person must be taken seriously and might include a history of the following:

  Theft or misappropriation of resources
  Enforced social isolation or confinement
  Threats or coercion

Use of restraints; locking in room
Battering
Sexual abuse
Threats of punishment
Withholding food, clothing, or privileges to enforce behavior

Although health care professionals will be more likely to observe the physical manifestations of abuse, they should try to elicit a history of other possible manifestations if the examination is suggestive of abuse or neglect. Referrals to health care professionals may also come from the police or from community legal or social service agencies. In these instances the issues of assessment are the same, although the types of cases may be different. The police are likely to see evidence of enforced confinement or be summoned to the scene by neighbors in the case of verbal abuse or threats of violence. Legal and social service agencies may see evidence of financial exploitation, especially when transfer of assets is undertaken.

The presence of any of these physical manifestations of inadequate care, including abuse and neglect, or a suggestive history, should trigger further evaluation by the health care professional in an attempt to identify any other potential areas of inadequate care.

RISK FACTORS FOR INADEQUATE CARE

There are groups of elderly persons who are at greater potential risk for abuse, neglect, or inadequate care than the population at large. A similar, detailed review is warranted for these people. Some of these high-risk groups are:

1. Those with chronic progressive, disabling illnesses that impair function and create care needs that exceed or will exceed their caretaker's ability to meet them, such as:

    a. Dementia
    b. Parkinsonism
    c. Severe arthritis
    d. Severe cardiac disease
    e. Severe COPD
    f. Severe AODM
    g. Recurrent strokes

2. Those with progressive impairments who are without informal supports from family or neighbors, or whose caretakers manifest signs of "burnout"
3. Those with a personal history of substance abuse or violent behavior or a family member or caretaker with same
4. Those who live with a family in which there is a history of child or spouse abuse
5. Those with family members who are financially dependent on them
6. Those residing in institutions that have a history of providing substandard care
7. Those whose caretakers are under sudden increased stress, due, for example, to loss of job, health, or spouse

It is important to note that these high-risk groups do not include socioeconomic parameters. This is because research to date has found cases of abuse and neglect in all social and economic strata, in rural and urban settings, in all religious groups, and in all races.

Even if elderly persons in these groups do not manifest any signs of inadequate care, it is useful to review in detail their activities of daily living and the extent and reliability of their caretaking help. Not only may such a review uncover actual unmet needs, but it might permit prospective intervention to avoid the development of an unmet need. The most effective time to intervene in these cases is before significant harm has occurred to the elderly person. Attention to these high-risk groups facilitates preventive intervention.

SCREENING INSTRUMENTS

Use of screening instruments is another strategy for identifying elderly persons who are likely to be receiving inadequate care, abuse, or neglect. Such instruments usually survey most of the items listed previously. In addition to identifying elderly persons who meet the criteria of inadequate care, these instruments provide a thorough data base for assessment. Unfortunately, screening instruments for the detection and assessment of elder abuse are few in number and subject to criticism based on a number of issues. First, since there are no universal definitions of elder abuse, neglect, or mistreatment, it is difficult to develop an instrument with wide applicability. Second, the clinical assessment of suspected elder abuse or neglect cases needs to remain in the "professional judgment" domain. It is only through experience that a health care provider can begin to discuss a typical presentation for elder abuse or neglect. However, the instruments to date serve the very useful functions of heightening professional awareness of the problem of elder abuse and guiding the clinician through a series of high-risk symptoms that could otherwise be missed. For these reasons, screening instruments should be encouraged as a regular feature of geriatric admissions and home visits.

A common approach suggested by several authors (Falconi, 1982; Ferguson & Beck, 1983; Phillips, 1983; Saunders & Plummer, 1983) has been the use of the standard review of systems in conjunction with guidelines such as those put forth by the U.S. Department of Health and Human Services (1980) of high-risk abuse situations. Another approach that is used in the study of elder abuse is the formation of categories of situations that appear to be associated with a high risk for abuse or neglect (Fulmer, 1984; Fulmer & Cahill, 1984; Fulmer, Street, & Carr, 1984; O'Malley, Everitt, O'Malley, & Campion, 1983). These categories are listed on the assessment instrument. The health care provider is then asked to rate the degree to which the category applies to the patient in question.

A problem with protocols is that they can be very lengthy and time consuming for the practitioner and may require more than one day for completion. However, the assessment is generally very thoroughly outlined and when conducted as directed is likely to provide conclusive information regarding the alleged abuse or neglect. Narrative reports are more cumbersome and less consistent in content than structured questionnaires.

THE ELDER ASSESSMENT INSTRUMENT

Given the aforementioned caveats of assessment instruments, let us now consider in detail an adaptation of a screening instrument currently in use (see Appendix A). Known as the Elder Assessment Instrument (EAI), it is used with patients in whom there is evidence of inadequate care, who are referred for specialized assessment. This instrument is given in its entirety in the following table, but a few words of explanation are in order first.

When performing an assessment with the EAI, information elicited should be detailed as well as discrete. The health care professional should obtain a baseline history, whenever possible, from the patient directly. In the case of confused patients, it will be necessary to obtain data from family, friends, current care providers, and old records, if they are available. Contact with these individuals should be initiated with discretion, especially when any of those individuals are suspected to have caused the condition under review. Questions are phrased in a nonaccusatory manner with an emphasis on clinical findings and descriptions of how the event or symptoms seemed to have occurred. The obvious sensitivity of the subject of abuse warrants an in-kind sensitivity in history taking.

General assessment parameters that help make the diagnosis of abuse, neglect, or mistreatment are organized into an approach that elicits information regarding these three categories. The EAI is organized to elicit clinical signs and symptoms, as perceived by the health care professional, upon assessment of the elderly person in question. The eight sections of the EAI have been formulated based on the background and theories for understanding elder abuse described in Chapter 2. Each of these sections is described in the text following Table 3-3.

Demographic Data

Information regarding the patient's age, sex, payment status, residence, mental status, and reason for the hospital visit are noted upon admission. For most elderly individuals it is likely that they are living in a private home setting and are accompanied by a family member or friend. In the case of elder abuse victims, it is not unusual for the elder to present at the hospital alone. Mental status assessment is important in order to determine if the history can be considered accurate. Documentation of mental status is also important due to the fact that the confused patient is considered to be a high-risk individual for abuse, neglect, or mistreatment. The reasons for the visit should be recorded in order to identify any pathophysiology that may be causing ambiguous clinical symptoms that may be misrepresented as abuse, neglect, or mistreatment.

General Assessment

General assessment parameters include attention to the individual's hygiene, nutrition, and clothing. As part of the initial observation, the health care professional assesses the hygiene of the patient and makes a notation stating who is responsible for the maintenance of the hygiene. In the case of many frail elders who live alone, it is not unusual for hygiene needs to be neglected due to failing vision, impaired mobility, and limiting chronic disorders. However, in the case of elders who are being cared for by others, it is reasonable to expect that some effort to maintain hygiene has been initiated. The assessment should reflect findings of lice, urine burns, smeared feces, or other obvious outstanding

TABLE 3-3 Elder Assessment Instrument (EAI)*

CONFIDENTIAL

1. DEMOGRAPHIC DATA

Date _____ Person Completing Form _____

Payment Status (Please check one):
____ Blue Cross/Blue Shield ____ Medicaid
____ Medicare ____ Private Payment ____ Other

Residence (Please check one):
____ Home _____ Name of Nursing Home
____ Other (e.g., son/daughter's home)

Accompanied by: ____ Family ____ Friend ____ Alone
____ Nursing Home Personnel

Reason for Visit: ____ Cardiac ____ Changed Mental Status
____ Fall ____ G.I. ____ Orthopedic
____ Other (please state) _____

Current Mental Status: ____ Oriented ____ Confused
____ Unresponsive

____ Age

2. GENERAL ASSESSMENT	Very good	Good	Undecided	Poor	Very poor	No basis for judgment
a. Clothing						
b. Hygiene						
c. Nutrition						
d. Skin integrity						

Additional Comments: _____
_____
_____
_____

*A revision of the instrument is again in progress.

TABLE 3-3 (Continued)

3. PHYSICAL ASSESSMENT	Definite evidence	Probable evidence	Uncertain	Probably no evidence	No evidence	No basis for judgment
a. Bruises						
b. Contractures						
c. Decubiti						
d. Dehydration						
e. Diarrhea						
f. Impaction						
g. Lacerations						
h. Malnutrition						
i. Urine burns/excoriations						

Additional Comments: _____

_____

_____

4. USUAL LIFESTYLE	Totally independent	Mostly independent	Uncertain	Mostly dependent	Totally dependent	No basis for judgment
a. Administration of medications						
b. Ambulation						
c. Continence						
d. Feedings						
e. Maintenance of hygiene						
f. Management of finances						
g. Family involvement						

TABLE 3–3 (*Continued*)

Additional Comments: _____

_____

_____

_____

5. SOCIAL ASSESSMENT

Narrative statement regarding patient-identified social problems: _____

_____

_____

Family/nursing home perception of problem: _____

_____

_____

_____

_____

	Very good quality	Good quality	Uncertain	Poor quality	Very poor quality	No basis for judgment
a. Financial situation						
b. Interaction with family						
c. Interaction with friends						
d. Interaction with nursing home personnel						
e. Living arrangement						
f. Observed relationship with care provider						
g. Participation in daily social activities						
h. Support systems						
i. Ability to express needs						

TABLE 3–3 (*Continued*)

Additional Comments (recent changes in life situation): ——————

——————————————————————————————

——————————————————————————————

——————————————————————————————

——————————————————————————————

6. MEDICAL ASSESSMENT	Definite evidence	Evidence	Possibility	Probably no evidence	No evidence	No basis/not applicable
a. Duplication of similar medications (e.g., multiple laxatives, sedatives)						
b. Unusual doses of medication						
c. Alcohol/substance abuse						
d. Greater than 15% dehydration						
e. Bruises and/or fractures beyond what is compatible with alleged trauma						
f. Failure to respond to warning of obvious disease						
g. Repetitive admissions due to probable failure of health care surveillance						

(Attach description of any additional physical findings) Additional comments (*Note*: if either 6a or 6b has been answered in the affirmative, please elaborate and be as specific as possible): ——————————

——————————————————————————————

——————————————————————————————

TABLE 3–3 (Continued)

	Definite evidence	Evidence	Possibility	Probably no evidence	No evidence	No basis/not applicable
7. SUMMARY ASSESSMENT						
a. Evidence of financial/ possession abuse						
b. Evidence of physical abuse						
c. Evidence of psychological abuse						
d. Evidence of neglect						

Additional Comments: _____

_____

_____

_____

	Yes	No
8. DISPOSITION		
a. Referral to elder assessment team		
b. Referral to clinical advisor		

General Comments (nursing home contact person and date):

_____

_____

_____

Summary statement in regard to abuse/neglect/mistreatment and follow-up plan:

_____

_____

TABLE 3-3 (Continued)

Date _____   _____ R.N.

                              _____ M.S.W.

                              _____ M.D.

Source: T. Fulmer, S. Street, & K. Carr. Abuse of the Elderly: Screening and Detection. *Journal of Emergency Nursing, 10* (May/June), 1984, 131–140. Reprinted with permission.

hygienic problems, as well as any possible causative factors for such a presentation.

Nutritional status, as an initial observation, can only reflect a judgment of the assessor in relation to the elder's physical stature, body weight, signs of dehydration; plus the patient's subjective comments regarding hunger and appetite. Due consideration to the elder's place of residence is obviously important. In the case of an elder who lives alone, poor nutrition may be the result of inadequate finances, transportation problems, or inadequate food storage or cooking facilities. For the elder who lives with a family member, it is reasonable to expect that nutritional needs are being met, as long as there is no evidence of anorexia or some other clinical disorder that leads to a cachectic state, such as advanced cancer. When the elder is presenting from a long-term-care facility, it is reasonable to expect that clinical indices of malnutrition are absent unless that is the reason for referral to the acute-care setting or unless there is documentation describing and explaining the current nutritional state of the patient.

The elder's clothing should be evaluated for its appropriateness to the current climate. Unsuitable dress may be the choice of the elder; however, it may also be due to inattention by a care provider.

Physical Assessment

Obvious symptoms of trauma must be reported to the physician and accurately recorded, and the cause must be clearly determined. Bilateral bruising, unexplained hematomas, or evidence of rope burns are examples of symptoms that need to be carefully assessed. The indicators that appear in Table 3-2 are all high-risk clinical symptoms and warrant careful review of causation. It may be important to obtain a specialty consult in order to provide a clear rationale for unusual injuries. For example, in the case of an unexplained hip fracture, it may take an orthopedic consult to determine if the elder's clinical state could engender a fracture without history of a fall or trauma. In a like manner, a decubitus ulcer of considerable size may need evaluation by a specialist in order to ascertain if the ulcer could have developed to its current extent and severity in spite of reasonable care, given an elder's physical condition. A 90-year-old patient with advanced cancer may present with a decubitus ulcer of equal size and pathology as that of a 60-year-old patient with a cerebral-vascular accident. It may be reasonable to expect different outcomes for each of these patients.

Usual Lifestyle

The assessment also obtains information regarding the elder's usual lifestyle, in order to get a clearer understanding of both the amount of physical care required and the elder's dependency needs. Information regarding assistance required for maintenance of hygiene, continence, feeding, and ambulation and management of finances and transportation modes is important. Douglass, Hickey, and Noele (1980) note that as dependency needs increase there appears to be a concommitant increase in elder abuse and neglect events, although this finding has not been replicated. They propose dependency as a hypothesis for why abuse events occur. Information regarding the elder's opportunity to get out, socialize, and remain active provides insight into the living situation. The possibility that the elder may also be dependent on the care provider for all social interaction should be explored.

Reports of any recent life crises need to be recorded, as there is also evidence to suggest that situational crises such as the loss of employment, divorce, death of a significant other, or legal problems may trigger an abuse event (Douglass et al. 1980).

Social Assessment

In order to obtain an accurate social assessment, the health care professional needs to recognize that there are limitations to an initial assessment. Only by developing a strategy for collecting more detailed information over time will an adequate social assessment be obtained. When elderly individuals are first screened in the acute-care setting, key questions to ask them relate to their self-identified social problems and their perception of their current life situation. The patient's value system may not be readily discernible. Over time, with the input of family and friends, a clearer social assessment usually emerges.

For the purpose of initial screening, it is useful to ask the patient broad questions that help identify potential problem areas. Since there is evidence to suggest that social isolation may be a factor in elder abuse, questions regarding the quality of interactions are helpful (Pillemer, 1984). There should be an assessment of interactions between the patient and family, friends, nursing home personnel, and home health aides, as appropriate.

Evidence of a lack of social support systems can suggest isolation for elders. This does not imply that all elders who are without social supports are victims, but it may provide insight into ineffective coping mechanisms.

Some elders have a difficult time expressing their needs and are not able to identify areas of concern. It may be necessary to rely more heavily on observational skills in these cases. If possible, it is useful to observe participation in social activities that serve as opportunities for validating the elder's social behavior, for observing norms among peers, and for noting lifestyles.

Financial assessments are important in order to get a sense of monetary stress or problems. At one end of the spectrum, an elder may have little or no financial reserve, which may trigger an abuse or neglect event if the stress is significant. At the other end of the spectrum, an elder who is well endowed financially may be in danger of victimization and exploitation by care providers. The elderly person may have handed over his or her financial management to a friend or relative and may not even be aware of unusual or unethical financial actions. It is also possible that an elderly person may feel that the only way to obtain help and services is by giving away money, possessions, or other sources of equity in order to maintain support from care providers. The possibility of robbery should be considered if an elderly individual is unable to account for a loss of funds or assets. There has been documentation of families who sell household furnishings and personal possessions of elders during acute hospitalizations, without the permission of the elder. Also, exploitation and victimization occur at both ends of the continuum. Some elders who only have Social Security checks as assets may also be exploited in that such checks may be used for family needs only, instead of the needs of the elder.

Medical Assessment

The assessment should also include, to the greatest extent possible, the number and type of medications the elder is currently taking, with documentation of the prescribed dosages. Evidence of duplication of similar medications, unusual dosages, or inadequate understanding of current medication regimens may explain an unusual clinical presentation. For example, an elder who utilizes multiple laxatives may be prone to altered fluid and electrolyte balance, weakness, dizziness, and falls. An elder with multiple prescriptions for sedatives may be given inappropriate dosages in order to provide respite time for tired or frustrated family members. Unknowing duplication of prescriptions may also result from fragmented health care. It is also possible that medication may be being withheld by care providers for the purpose of usurping those medications for their own use. If the assessor feels this is a possibility, it should be brought to the attention of the prescribing physician immediately so that the appropriate interventions can be made. When elders misunderstand their medication regimen, dire consequences can result which may be misinterpreted as abuse. Health care interventions including medication teaching, special delivery systems such as numbered containers, and community nursing referrals can prevent any further occurrence.

Other items under the medical assessment include alcohol/substance abuse and dehydration. Both of these can be substantiated through laboratory values. Items E, F, and G require clinical decisionmaking relative to whether an elderly person presents in a manner that is inconsistent with the alleged story or incompatible with the level of care that may be expected given the site the elder is coming from. Additional comments are encouraged under this section, which are extremely useful in clarifying any of the items that are checked off as being in evidence.

Summary Assessments

Obviously, an accurate and tactful elder abuse assessment takes time. Whenever there seems to be an indication of an unusual circumstance in any of the previous subcategories, an in-depth assessment should follow. It is important to encourage health professionals to discuss possible abuse, neglect, or mistreatment with an appropriate hospital resource person, such as an administrator, lawyer, physician, or social worker. The first step in understanding these events comes from discussing concerns with colleagues. Whenever there is a possibility that elder abuse has occurred, a high level of suspicion is warranted until there is a reasonable explanation.

Disposition

The disposition section of the EAI documents where the referral has been made and provides space for comment and follow-up. This section becomes particularly useful when reviewing past cases for outcomes and for following patients longitudinally. At the Beth Israel Hospital, a system has been put in place whereby all patients who are referred for suspected abuse to the hospital's Elder Assessment Team are "flagged" during subsequent admissions by a notation that appears by the patient's unit number each time they are readmitted to the hospital. It is a very subtle notation that does not draw attention to the patient unless staff are instructed to look for it. It is the emergency unit staff and elder assessment team members who are so instructed.

RESULTS FROM THE BETH ISRAEL HOSPITAL STUDY

The Elder Assessment Instrument (EAI) has served as a valuable data-collection instrument for patients referred to the Beth Israel Hospital Elder Assessment Team. Over time, data collected have been tallied in order to provide insight into who gets referred to the Elder Assessment Team and why (Fulmer & Cahill, 1984).

Over the past five years at Beth Israel Hospital, 108 cases have been referred to the Elder Assessment Team for suspicion of abuse, neglect, or mistreatment. Three pilot studies conducted in the emergency unit (see Appendix A) have assessed all presenting elders over the age of 70 years, not merely those referred to the abuse team, in order to develop the EAI to its current format and provide a baseline compar-

TABLE 3–4 Pilot Studies for the EAI

Pilot 1: August 1981	161 elders over 70 years of age assessed with EAI #1
Pilot 2: April 1982– August 1982	484 elders over 70 years of age assessed with EAI #2
Pilot 3: February 1983	146 elders over 70 years of age assessed with EAI #3

ison group (see Table 3–4). For the purpose of improving the elder assessment instrument clinically, the format labels and scoring methods have changed after each study period, which precludes the possibility of comparing data from the three different time periods except in the most general way. Therefore, only data from the third pilot have been used as a "comparison group" with the elder abuse referral group.

Each assessment item on the EAI is ranked from 1 (positive) to 5 (negative). Utilizing mean scores for each item in comparing the cases referred to the Elder Assessment Team with those from the February 1983 comparison group, it is possible to note differences between the two. The results are shown in Table 3–5.

TABLE 3–5 Emergency Unit Comparison Group versus Elder Abuse Referral Group

Variable	Comparison Group (N = 146)	Elder Abuse Referral Group (N = 108)	χ^2
Mean age:	80.9	82.7	$p < .05$
Residence (%):			$p < .001$
Own home	75	36	
Nursing home	19	45	
Other	5	19	

(Continued)

TABLE 3–5 (Continued)

Variable	Comparison Group (N = 146)	Elder Abuse Referral Group (N = 108)	χ^2
Accompanied by (%):			$p < .001$
Family	50	24	
Friend	4	2	
Alone	44	73	
Nursing home personnel	1	3	
Reason for visit (%):			$p < .05$
Cardiac	18	6	
Changed mental status	8	13	
Fall	20	23	
G.I.	6	3	
Orthopedic	4	11	
Other (respiratory or sepsis)	44	44	
Mental status (%):			$p < .001$
Oriented	85	29	
Confused	12	56	
Unresponsive	5	15	
General assessment (mean score):			
Clothing	1.8	3.0	$p < .001$
Hygiene	1.7	3.0	$p < .001$
Nutrition	1.9	3.4	$p < .001$
Skin	1.9	3.4	$p < .001$
Physical assessment (mean score):			
Bruising	1.5	2.9	$p < .001$
Contractures	1.3	2.3	$p < .001$
Decubuti	1.2	2.8	$p < .001$
Dehydration	1.4	2.9	$p < .001$
Diarrhea	1.3	1.7	$p < .01$
Impaction	1.1	2.0	$p < .001$
Lacerations	1.2	1.9	$p < .001$
Malnutrition	1.1	2.4	$p < .001$
Urine burns	1.1	1.7	$p < .001$
Usual lifestyle (mean score):			
Administration of medications	2.4	4.1	$p < .001$
Ambulation	2.0	3.5	$p < .001$
Continence	1.7	3.3	$p < .001$
Feedings	1.7	3.1	$p < .001$
Maintenance of hygiene	1.9	3.6	$p < .001$
Management of finances	2.4	3.8	$p < .001$
Family involvement	n.a.[a]	3.3	

TABLE 3–5 (Continued)

Variable	Comparison Group (N = 146)	Elder Abuse Referral Group (N = 108)	χ^2
Social assessment (mean score):			
Financial situation	2.3	3.3	$p < .001$
Interaction with family	2.1	3.1	$p < .001$
Interaction with friends	2.7	3.2	$p < .001$
Interaction with nursing home personnel	2.7	2.7	n.s.[b]
Living arrangement	1.9	3.3	$p < .001$
Observed relationship with careprovider	2.4	3.0	$p < .01$
Participation in social activities	2.6	3.5	$p < .001$
Support systems	n.a.	3.1	
Ability to express needs	n.a.	4.0	
Medical assessment (mean score):			
Duplication of medications	1.1	1.1	n.s.
Unusual doses of medications	1.1	1.2	n.s.
Alcohol/substance abuse	1.1	1.3	n.s.
Greater than 15% dehydration	n.a.	3.9	
Bruises/fractures beyond what is compatible with trauma	n.a.	4.4	
Failure to respond to warning signals of obvious disease	n.a.	3.7	
Repetitive admissions	n.a.	4.3	
Summary assessments (mean score):			
Evidence of financial or possession abuse	1.2	1.4	$p < .05$
Evidence of physical abuse	1.1	2.8	$p < .001$
Evidence of psychological abuse	1.2	2.8	$p < .001$
History of recent life crisis	1.4	2.2	$p < .01$

[a]n.a. = not available (no such item on list at time of pilot study).
[b]n.s. = not significant.

Both groups are very old (mean age is over 75 years), but, due to the selection process of the comparison group (over 70 years of age), no specific comments can be made except to note the very old mean age of the elder abuse referral group. Referrals generally are made for patients who live in nursing homes ($p < .001$), come in alone ($p < .001$), and are assessed as "confused" ($p < .001$). Therefore, it appears that there is a relationship between these variables and the incidence of referral to the Elder Assessment Team. The large percentage of nursing home referrals may be due to the older age and greater dependency of elders in nursing homes in general. A good number of this nursing home group arrives at the hospital alone via ambulance. The elders who present "alone" may be referred more often due to a lack of an advocacy figure accompanying them, and the confused elder may also be referred more often because it is not possible to obtain a history and account for signs and symptoms.

There also appears to be a difference between mean item scores for the two groups in that the comparison group tends to receive a more positive score on the instrument assessment items than the elder abuse referral group. It appears that those patients who are most likely to be referred to the Elder Assessment Team are likely to receive a poorer rating on the general assessment presentation related to clothing, hygiene, nutrition, and skin condition. They are also more likely to have some evidence of the items noted under the physical assessment section, such as bruising, contractures, decubiti, or dehydration; and they are noted to be more dependent in terms of the items listed under the "usual lifestyle" section. The social assessment section reveals that they are less interactive with significant others, and the medical assessment section does not indicate any significant differences between the two groups. Other items in the medical assessment category cannot be commented on, as they were added after the third pilot study, although comparisons will be possible in the future.

The profiles of the two groups must be reviewed with two caveats in mind: (1) Since the profile is based on mean scores, individual patients may deviate greatly, particularly in areas where standard deviations associated with the means are large, and (2) most elderly patients who come to an emergency room unit either are independent and alert enough to present themselves for treatment or have individuals who care enough about them to bring them in for treatment, with the exception of those who come by ambulance.

CREATING A RESPONSIBLE PROCESS FOR HANDLING ABUSE CASES

Assessments compiled over time at Beth Israel indicate a trend among those referred to the Elder Assessment Team to present with symptoms of confusion, dehydration, incontinence, fractures, and skin breakdown. It is important to ask ourselves whether these individuals are more "at risk" for referral because of the underlying inadequate care that can cause this constellation of symptoms or because we are confusing elder abuse and neglect with common pathology in the aged. While two individuals may present with equal fractures or equal decubiti, if the care provider clearly indicates concern regarding the elder's health, there is less chance that the situation will be labeled abuse. When the care provider indicates a lack of concern, an abuse label is much more likely (Phillips, 1983).

We propose that "risk factors," as we currently understand them, need further refinement. The variables listed in the EAI do trigger referrals from clinicians who are concerned for the well-being and safety of the elderly they are caring for (see Figure 3-1). It seems prudent, given the limited knowledge we have about elder abuse, to develop in-house reporting systems that allow cases to be reviewed before they reach the state agency level. This may prevent

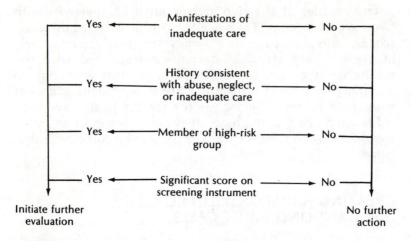

FIGURE 3-1 Clues to the potential for or presence of abuse, which trigger successive steps in case management.

accusations from being made before enough information is obtained, which serves as a protective mechanism for the elderly in that it diminishes the likelihood of premature or inappropriate disruption in their place of residence. It is extremely important to have a consistent process for handling elder abuse cases, for the safety of the patient.

There are limits to intervention which must be recognized. It is important to realize that the elderly person's right to refuse any assessment or intervention extends to issues concerning abuse, neglect, or inadequate care. Unless a court determines that an elderly person is incompetent to act in his or her own best interests and appoints a guardian, there is the presumption that the elderly person alone can determine what is appropriate and acceptable intervention. Unlike child abuse, in which the government assumes the right to intervene on the child's behalf, thereby overruling the parents, in cases of elder abuse the elderly person determines the goals of intervention. In a sense there is a right to be abused which must be respected. However, as health professionals, an ethical obligation exists to assure that if such a right is exercised, it is without coercion and with full knowledge of the alternatives.

SUMMARY

Health care professionals should seek evidence for inadequate care as part of the evaluation of any elderly person presenting for medical or psychosocial evaluation. By examining the patient for manifestations of abuse, neglect, and inadequate care; by actively trying to elicit history suggestive of abuse or neglect; and by noting that the patient is a member of a high-risk group, the health care professional can take an active role in the early identification of these cases. Particular attention should be paid to the assessment of members of the high-risk groups.

REFERENCES

Douglass, R. C., Hickey, T., & Noele, C. (1980). *A Study of Maltreatment of the Elderly and Other Vulnerable Adults*. Ann Arbor, MI: University of Michigan, Institute of Gerontology.

Falconi, D. (1982). Assessing the Abused Elderly. *Journal of Gerontological Nursing, 8*(4), 208–212.

Ferguson, D., & Beck, C. (1983, September/October). H.A.L.F.—A Tool to Assess Elder Abuse within the Family. *Geriatric Nursing*, 301–304.

Fulmer, T. (1984). Elder Abuse Assessment Tool. *Dimension of Critical Care Nursing, 3*(4), 216–220.

Fulmer, T., & Cahill, V. (1984). Elder Abuse: A Study. *Journal of Gerontological Nursing, 10*(12), 16–20.

Fulmer, T., Street, S., & Carr, K. (1984, May/June). Abuse of the Elderly: Screening and Detection. *Journal of Emergency Nursing, 10,* 131–140.

O'Malley, T., Everitt, D., O'Malley, H., & Campion, E. (1983). Identifying and Preventing Family-Mediated Abuse and Neglect of Elderly Persons. *Annals of Internal Medicine, 98*(6, Part 2), 998–1005.

Phillips, L. R. (1983, May/June). Elder Abuse—What Is It?–Who Says So? *Geriatric Nursing*, 167–170.

Pillemer, K. (1984). The Dangers of Dependency: New Findings on Domestic Violence against the Elderly. Unpublished manuscript.

Rathbone-McCuan, E., & Voyles, B. (1982). Case Detection of Abuse of Elderly Patients. *American Journal of Psychiatry, 139*, 189–192.

Saunders, F. V., & Plummer, E. M. (1983, July). Assault on the Aged: Is Your Patient a Secret Victim? *RN*, 21–25.

U.S. Department of Health and Human Services. (1980, May). *Family Violence: Intervention Strategies*. Human Development Series, DHHS Pub. No. (OHDS) 80-30258. Washington, DC: U.S. Government Printing Office.

4

Gaining Access to
Those in Need

Elder abuse has been called the "hidden problem" of domestic violence. Gaining access to the elderly person who is receiving inadequate care for any reason can be extremely difficult. In this section we will consider the various problems practitioners face in trying to reach those in need, and the strategies they use to overcome these problems. In each of these categories of elderly persons, we are assuming that reports suggesting the possibility of inadequate care have come to the attention of the health care professional.

We include under the problems of access both physical and interpersonal barriers that prevent adequate assessment and intervention. Access can be limited by the elderly person, by caretakers (both family and neighbors), and by institutions. In the early studies on abuse and neglect of the elderly at home, access was not possible in up to 40 percent of the cases selected for further assessment (O'Malley, Segars, & Perez, 1979). Failure to gain access made assessment and intervention impossible. As might be imagined, it is extremely difficult to study these individuals and families in order to ascertain if they share any common characteristics that might explain why they refused access or intervention. We will discuss three groups of elderly persons: those who live alone, those who live with family, and those living in institutions. Each presents a different set of problems.

ACCESS TO ELDERS WHO LIVE ALONE

Elderly persons who live alone at home and are receiving inadequate care present a commonly encountered problem that unfortunately falls outside of the perview of most abuse and neglect statutes. These individuals are likely to come to the attention of the health care system because of a report by a neighbor, friend, landlord, clergy, or other individual who has the opportunity to call on the elderly person at home. They also may be brought to a physician or hospital for evaluation and treatment of a medical or psychological problem that those members of their support system deem significant. In the latter case, the problem of physically gaining access to the elderly person is at least temporarily absent, and a large part of the barrier to evaluation and intervention is removed because the elderly person has already accepted the advice (however reluctantly) to seek medical care.

Although the chances of assessment and intervention are significantly greater in this situation, several barriers persist and can effectively block any intervention. Although these barriers are internal to the individual, they are no less important than physical barriers such as distance and lack of resources. They include the following:

1. Fear of loss of autonomy
2. Fear of financial burden
3. Embarrassment
4. Concern for privacy
5. Desire to be left alone
6. Fear of change
7. Stigma of accepting social service or mental health care

8. Distrust of doctors, nurses, social workers, large institutions
9. Skepticism regarding the efficacy of medical/social interventions
10. Cognitive disorders such as paranoia, dementia, and depression
11. Inability to make decisions

It is important to recognize at the outset that it is the elderly person's prerogative to end any discussion regarding his or her care at any time. The health care professional must lay the groundwork for a future relationship as quickly as possible, while still gathering the information necessary to prevent further harm to the elderly person. If the initial contact does not lead to subsequent contacts, however restricted, then the opportunity to intervene has been lost until the next crisis occurs. In the meantime the elderly person is exposed to the risk of further harm.

We have found the following approach to be an effective way to initiate the evaluation of individuals who are brought into the medical, mental health, and social service systems, either voluntarily or at the insistence of a third party; it does not matter if the elderly person lives alone, with family, or in an institution. It involves the following three steps.

Step 1: Opening Communication

An immediate attempt should be made to identify the elderly person's response to the *process* of assessment—whether it is positive or negative. If negative, listen to the concerns the elderly person has about the process. This can be accomplished by responding to the nonverbal and verbal clues that the elderly person gives when the health care professional introduces himself or herself. We have found that statements such as the following are an effective way to begin an interview: "My name is _____; I work for

_____. I apologize for any difficulty this has caused you. I can understand how this could make you _____ (angry, nervous, uncomfortable, sad, scared, etc.)." This usually evokes some comment from the elderly person, to which the health care professional can react. Initially, it is usually easier for the elderly person to talk about the process of being interviewed than it is to answer direct questions about personal issues. The health care professional can then proceed to work through the elderly person's feelings about involving an outsider in personal concerns. With this opening statement, the health care professional conveys several important messages: respect for the feelings of the elderly person, willingness to treat the person as an individual, and the ability to understand the person's point of view. This helps to remove concerns that might impede further discussion if not addressed and removed at the outset.

Step 2: Reviewing Activities of Daily Living

An attempt should be made to ascertain the elderly person's care needs by reviewing a typical day, with particular attention to how individual ADL's are accomplished (see Chapter 5). It is important to explain why this information is necessary and to emphasize that this is a process over which the elderly person has control. Many elderly persons are reluctant or embarrassed to discuss their problems with toileting, hygiene, or dressing. A less threatening approach to information gathering is to seek evidence of significant disabilities by asking questions that suggest that difficulties are the norm rather than the exception, thereby putting the elderly person at ease. For example, you might say, "Some things are more easily done than others, and most people have difficulty with something. Are there any activities that cause you a little difficulty, like climbing stairs, using a phone?" Move from the least sensitive issues like shopping or preparing meals to dressing, bathing, and toileting. Unless the elderly person volunteers information about who helps or doesn't help, such information is best left for later, because it may represent an emotionally charged issue that the elderly person will resist discussing.

Step 3: Clarifying Priorities

Attempt to clarify the elderly person's priorities among potential choices such as safety, comfort, and remaining at home. You might ask, "Would you want to stay in your own apartment, even if you could be safer or more comfortable living with family or friends?" Be ready to shift to a different, less emotionally charged topic if the elderly person shows reluctance to discuss this: "You don't have to talk about that if you don't want to."

These initial steps in the interview are critical. Time is better spent identifying and relieving the elderly person's concerns than pursuing the health care professional's agenda of gathering information. Even in such a limited interview, valuable information can be gained about the elderly person's emotional well-being, cognitive ability, and perception of illness or disability. If this process is interrupted by the elderly person, the health care professional should try to arrange a definite follow-up interview, in order to continue the assessment.

For the elderly person who lives alone at home and who is to be seen at home, not at the hospital or agency, the same approach applies. In addition, however, there are two techniques which have proved helpful in getting through the front door. The first is to have the initial meeting scheduled by a friend or family member of the elderly person, and if possible have that person present during the start of the interview. Until the health care professional and the elderly person establish a relationship, the presence of a trusted friend makes the elderly person less resistant to the questioning.

If that is not possible, then an attempt must be made to

make the initial encounter as nonthreatening as possible. We have found that the visiting nurses and home care agency staff are more successful than mental health or social service workers in gaining access for an initial assessment. Their presence in the community is usually well known, and they have a reputation for helping the elderly. They are nonthreatening and do not provoke in the elderly person the defensive reaction that the mere mention of "mental health" occasionally does. Just as important, however, they can convincingly explain the purpose of their visit to be a "survey of services which might be needed for elderly in the neighborhood," which is an effective stratagem. Physicians, too, are usually admitted if they have a prior relationship with the elderly person or are brought in by someone that the elderly person trusts.

Having gained access (by whatever means are effective), the health care professional follows the guidelines listed earlier for the initial interview.

ACCESS TO ELDERS WHO LIVE WITH FAMILY

The elderly person living at home with family presents a different set of issues. This situation is more complex because it involves at least two individuals, the elderly person and the family member who is the responsible caretaker. The least difficult scenario occurs when the elderly person is brought in for medical treatment. That provides the opportunity to establish a justification for further visits to the elderly person at home, making access for further assessment easier.

The most difficult situation, however, occurs when both the caretaker and the elderly person are resistant to "outside interference." Not only may the caretaker share the elderly person's reasons for not wanting anyone to become involved in a "family matter," but they may also resist the discovery of inadequate care to which they have contributed.

The most (but not universally) successful approach has been to address the concerns and needs of the caretaker prior to assessing those of the elder. In order to have a positive impact on the care of the elderly person, the health care professional must gain access to the elderly person. In order to gain access, the health care professional must gain the support and trust of the caretaker, who is usually the one who controls access to the elderly person. This can be done using the same sympathetic approach that was applied to the reluctant elder living alone.

Three points must be conveyed to the caretaker. The first is that no one is attempting to judge the quality of the caretaking efforts. The second is that the health care professional recognizes the difficulties that the caretaker has faced to provide care and that sacrifices have been made. And finally, the professional must affirm that the caretaking role is a valuable one and cannot be easily replaced. These points are not only appreciated by the caretaker but they also represent the correct attitude for the health care professional to take. It takes a tremendous effort to meet all of the care needs of a functionally impaired elderly person. The health care professional needs to approach the caretaker by recognizing the effort involved in caring for an elderly parent. This can form the basis for a supportive relationship between the caretaker and the health care professional.

We have found it helpful to use the following approach: "We know how difficult it is to take care of an elderly parent. Your time is not your own, and you can feel like you're being pulled in all directions at once. It's enough to make you feel like you're going to go crazy. Who is taking care of you?" This usually leads to a discussion of what the caretaker needs. If the caretaker perceives the role of the health care professional as supportive rather than judgmental or accusative, then the caretaker is more likely to permit ongoing involvement by the health care professional.

The transition to the assessment of the needs of the elderly person can usually be made in the following manner:

"One of the ways that we can help you (the caretaker) is to see if there aren't things that can be done for your parent to make it less difficult for you." This approach has been successful in some cases of "active neglect" and "abuse." Having worked through the resistance of the caretaker, the health care professional needs to do the same with the elderly person. By focusing on the nonjudgmental issues of "care needs," the professional helps the elderly person to avoid any implied criticism of the caretaker. It is difficult to maintain this attitude if one is looking for abuse and neglect rather than for inadequate care.

It is always preferable to use a nonjudgmental, supportive approach to gaining access. Not only is it more effective, but it also helps to maintain or strengthen the caretaking role of the family member. It may be difficult to replace this person, even though their efforts are inadequate or even counterproductive. By defining abuse and neglect as a crime, with a victim and a perpetrator, it is very difficult to focus on the care needs of the elderly person or on the positive aspects of the caretaker's actions. But by focusing on inadequate care rather than "abuse and neglect," the health care professional can more easily support the positive aspects of the caretaker's behavior and encourage new, more productive behavior.

It is occasionally necessary to gain access to an elderly person by force, using the police. It is important to recognize at the outset that, as a consequence of this approach, a negotiated relationship between the caretaker and the health care professional will, in all probability, never occur. It is also likely that the elderly person will resist any immediate steps to leave or to remove the caretaker. Only rarely will such an intervention result in any positive benefit for the elderly person. The usual result is to embarrass or anger the caretaker and the elderly person, thereby making them more resistant to outside contact. It also leaves the elderly person open to retaliation by the caretaker.

There is one circumstance in which this approach is effective. When the elderly person is incompetent and is receiving inadequate care for any reason, then forced entry offers one of the few means of bringing such individuals to the attention of the courts. If a competency hearing finds that the elderly person is not competent, then the court will appoint a guardian to supervise the care of the elderly person, under strict guidelines. In such a manner the future adequate care of the elderly person can be assured. (The issue of competency is discussed in more detail in Chapter 5; the ethical issues that are raised by nonvoluntary participation in a care plan are examined in Chapter 8.)

ACCESS TO INSTITUTIONALIZED ELDERS

The issues of access to elderly persons living in institutions are less problematic than with those living alone or with family. Most states have assumed the responsibility for assuring minimum standards of care for institutionalized elders. Medicare and Medicaid participants require frequent audits of services. Unfortunately, many of these audits emphasize paperwork compliance with state and federal regulations rather than assessment of the adequacy of the actual care received by the elderly person. As a result, systematic undertreatment of nursing home residents can and does go undetected and unreported. Access to these patients, however, can always be achieved through the appropriate state regulatory agency.

SUMMARY

The tasks of establishing access to the elderly person should take precedence over the process of assessment. Time taken initially to allay the concerns of the elderly person or caretaker may make the difference between successful intervention and total resistance to intervention. The key is to pay close attention to the fears and concerns of the elderly person and caretaker regarding the process of assessment and to promote the goal of resolving unmet care needs rather than the goal of identifying abuse or neglect.

REFERENCE

O'Malley, H. C., Segars, H. D., & Perez, R. (1979). *Elder Abuse in Massachusetts: A Survey of Professionals and Paraprofessionals.* Boston: Legal Research and Services for the Elderly.

5

Assessment

The issues of access merge into the issues of assessment once the elderly person's initial resistance to being interviewed is overcome. In order of priority, the principal tasks of assessment are:

1. Rapidly identify all unmet care needs that pose an immediate and significant threat to the elderly person's health; that is, assess the risk of imminent harm. Initiate action to protect the person if a significant risk exists.
2. Assess the person's level of competency.
3. Identify all significant care needs and potential needs (the person's functional status and health status) and determine the intensity of services required to meet them.
4. Identify the resources available to meet these needs and assess their stability and reliability.
5. Explore the possibility that the caretaker (if any) or other individual is contributing to care needs.
6. Identify the elderly person's priorities for intervention.

In this chapter each of these tasks will be discussed.

DETERMINING WHEN IMMEDIATE INTERVENTION IS NECESSARY

The initial assessment screens for imminent harm and determines the pace and urgency of intervention. Its purpose is to determine whether immediate interventions are required to prevent further harm to the elderly person. There are three circumstances requiring immediate action:

The presence of life-threatening medical problems
The presence of an unsafe environment
The presence of an individual with unimpeded access to the elderly person who has seriously harmed the elderly person in the past

It is relatively easy to determine the presence of life-threatening or serious medical problems on the basis of observation of the elderly person. In general these are acute rather than chronic conditions which severely compromise the elderly person's ability to function. The following acute problems should trigger an attempt to obtain a more complete medical evaluation:

Extreme confusion, delirium, or altered mental status
Evidence of profuse bleeding
Inability to walk or transfer
Inability to eat or drink
Signs of head trauma
Deformity indicating possible fracture
Indications of acute illness, such as fever, shortness of breath, hemiparesis, cellulitis, or dehydration

The presence of any of these acute conditions places the elderly person at extreme risk of death or further harm. These problems usually require evaluation in an emergency room and frequently require hospitalization.

The lack of heat, water, or food requires rapid intervention, which may range from removing the elderly person from the unsafe conditions to correcting those conditions. The elderly's inability to make sound judgments because of impaired sensation, blindness, confusion, or dementia may convert an otherwise safe environment into a potentially dangerous one. Stairs, gas stoves, and heaters may cause serious accidents if the elder requires supervision but it is not available. A prior history of fires, burns, or serious falls would be sufficient to make rapid intervention prudent.

The third source of potential harm is any individual who has threatened or actually harmed the elderly person. It may be extremely difficult to assess the validity of claims of beating or assault. It is also unlikely that the elder will admit that they have been harmed by a caretaker, especially if the caretaker is a family member. If reliable reports exist of serious harm at the hands of an individual with unimpeded access to the elderly person, then timely steps are required to separate the elder from the source of the threatened harm. This can be done by arranging for the elder to move in with other family or friends, to an emergency shelter; by moving someone else in with the elder who can provide protection; by restricting access to the elder by physical means such as new door locks; or by placing legal sanctions on the abuser by obtaining an emergency court order.

It is often easier to use the need for medical evaluation as an excuse to remove an elderly person from an unsafe environment or from potential exposure to physical abuse than to confront these issues directly. The advantages, disadvantages, and likelihood that the elderly person will accept these interventions are discussed in the next chapter. Suffice it to say that arranging for emergency care, shelter, or relocation requires skillful negotiation with the client and a command of the available emergency resources. Assessment and intervention proceed together when there is a risk of imminent harm.

If a threat of imminent harm exists and the health care professional can successfully negotiate an intervention with the elderly person, then further assessment can take place after the urgent care needs are met. If the client refuses interventions despite urgently needed care or protection, the health care professional faces a difficult conflict between two important issues, the right of the client to self-determination and the duty of the health care professional to provide necessary services. This dilemma is discussed in Chapter 8.

ASSESSING COMPETENCY

It is important to evaluate the elderly person's level of competency early in the process of assessment. Competency is the ability to make decisions and to understand the consequences and implications of those decisions. It is the ability to make sound judgments on the basis of available information. Intervention is a very different matter if the elderly person is found to be incompetent, since development of an intervention plan would be done with a court-appointed guardian and not necessarily with the client.

It is important to distinguish between incompetent decisions and irrational ones. An incompetent decision is one made by an individual who is unable to understand the consequences or significance of a decision. An irrational decision is one that makes no sense to us but is made by an individual who understands and accepts its consequences.

The competent person has the right to refuse any and all interventions. This has been upheld in several court decisions dealing with the right to refuse life-saving medical treatment. The courts have also upheld the right to remain in an abusive situation that poses the potential for significant harm (Lane *v*. Candura, 1978). In a sense, there is a "right to be abused," if the individual is competent and elects to exercise that right. An irrational decision does not indicate incompetency and is not grounds for attempting to restrict any person's freedom to make his or her own decisions. It is, however, a great source of concern and frustration for the health care professional.

In assessing competency, it is the process of decision making that requires scrutiny rather than the outcome. As noted already, an elderly person may arrive at a decision with which we disagree but which is in keeping with the priorities which he or she has set. If the person is able to justify the decision on the basis of some perceived benefit and is aware of the risks that such a decision might entail, then it is likely to be a competent decision. On the other hand, if the individual is confused, with poor short-term memory and other signs of dementia, then there is reason to question competency. The "mini mental exam" developed by Folstein, Folstein, & McHugh (1975) is a rapid means by which to assess the presence of dementia, a major cause of incompetency. A modified questionnaire based on their work is presented in Table 5-1.

It is important to realize that the courts have very specific definitions of incompetency which are usually very difficult to establish without expert testimony at a competency hearing. Throughout this process, the elderly person is assumed to be competent and the burden of proof is on those who would have the person judged incompetent. In addition, many courts recognize different levels of competency and respond with a decision that preserves the greatest level of independent functioning for the elderly person. A conservator may be named; this is a court-appointed person who has financial oversight and control and who is responsible for seeing that the elderly person's assets are used in that person's best interests. A guardianship represents the total control of the elderly person's assets and person. All decisions are made by the guardian on behalf of the elderly person, including life-and-death medical decisions.

Many state laws permit the health care professional to obtain an expedited decision regarding competency and an emergency decree permitting emergency intervention in life-threatening situations in which the elderly person is

TABLE 5–1 Mini Mental State Exam

Patient _____

Examiner _____

Date _____

Maximum Score	Score	
		Orientation:
5	( )	What is the (year) (season) (date) (day) (month)?
5	( )	Where are we (state) (county) (town) (hospital) (floor)?
		Registration:
3	( )	Name 3 objects: 1 second to say each. Then ask the patient all 3 after you have said them. Give 1 point for each correct answer. Then repeat them until he learns all 3. Count trials and record. Trials _____
		Attention and Calculation:
5	( )	Serial 7's: 1 point for each correct. Stop after 5 answers. Alternately, spell "world" backwards.
		Recall:
3	( )	Ask for 3 objects repeated above. Give 1 point for each correct answer.

cont.

thought to be incompetent to protect his or her own safety or well-being. These determinations are temporary and restricted and are not substitutes for full competency hearings.

IDENTIFYING SIGNIFICANT CARE NEEDS

The foundation of our approach to abuse and neglect is to identify the elderly person's unmet needs for care. Care needs are determined by three factors:

Physical disability
Psychological or cognitive disability
Environmental hazards

TABLE 5-1 (*Continued*)

			Language:
2	(	)	Name a pencil and watch (2 points)
1	(	)	Repeat the following: "no ifs, ands or buts" (1 point)
3	(	)	Follow a 3-stage command: "Take a paper in your right hand, fold it in half, and put it on the floor." (3 points)
1	(	)	Read and obey the following: "Close your eyes." (1 point)
1	(	)	Write a sentence (Must contain subject and verb and be sensible). (1 point)
			Visual-Motor Integrity:
1	(	)	Copy design (2 intersecting pentagons. All 10 angles must be present and 2 must intersect). (1 point)
_____			TOTAL SCORE _____
30			Assess level of consciousness along a continuum:

Alert	Drowsy	Stupor	Coma

Scoring: > 29 = normal, 22–27 = mild impairment, 18–22 = moderate impairment, < 18 = severe impairment.

Source: Adapted from M. F. Folstein, S. E. Folstein, & P. R. McHugh, Mini-Mental Method for Grading the Cognitive State of Patients for the Clinician. *Journal of Psychiatric Research, 12,* 189–198, 1975. © 1975, Pergamon Press, Ltd. Used with permission.

It is useful to consider each of these factors separately when assessing the elderly person's need for care, as each category requires a different approach.

Physical Disability

Use of functional status questionnaires is essential for consistent and complete evaluation of physical disabilities experienced by the elderly person. These disabilities, in turn, create the potential for care needs by limiting the elderly's capacity to provide self-care. Many functional status questionnaires exist and have been extensively and critically reviewed (Kane & Kane, 1981). The choice of a functional status tool is determined by the goals of the assessment, the

resources and personnel available to use it, and the population of elderly persons with whom it is being used. The
reader is referred to Kane and Kane for further discussion
of factors that must be considered in choosing an assessment tool. We have included in Appendix B a copy of the
Assessment and Functional Evaluation Form from the Massachusetts Elder Protective Services Program.

At a minimum the functional assessment should include
an evaluation of the following activities of daily living:

Use of the telephone	Eating
Traveling beyond walking	Dressing
distance	Grooming
Shopping	Walking
Preparing meals	Getting in and out of
Doing housework	bed
Taking medicine	Bathing
Managing finances	Toileting

Difficulty in performing any of these activities creates real
or potential needs for additional assistance. All have implications for various types of interventions.

Psychological or Cognitive Disability

Cognitive and psychological disabilities have significant impact on the elderly person's need for care. Cognitive disabilities can be formally assessed using the Mini Mental Status
Exam, however, the interviewer usually is able to assess the
presence of cognitive disabilities during the interview. Furthermore, description of the elderly person's ability to function, level of orientation, and degree of confusion can be
obtained from neighbors and friends who have observed the
elderly person. Prior history of hospitalization or treatment
for depression or psychosis and the current and past use of
psychotropic medications also provide clues to psychological
or cognitive impairment.

The presence of cognitive impairment creates several difficulties. The first is that it puts into question the validity

and accuracy of any historical data obtained from the elderly person. The interviewer must then rely more heavily on other sources of information. Having clarified the nature of the unmet needs for care, the health care professional must develop a more elaborate plan in order to compensate for the elderly person's inability to cooperate or understand the care plan. Confusion or forgetfulness on the part of the elderly person may contribute to an unsafe environment. An example would be forgetting to turn off a gas stove.

In addition, the evaluation of physical disabilities must include a thorough medical evaluation to identify health problems that currently result in disability or may cause or exacerbate a disability. The identification and treatment of inadequately managed medical problems is an essential part of intervention in managing cases of inadequate care. Medical problems may provide the "excuse" for more extensive home supports and monitoring of situations in which the elderly person is at risk for physical abuse.

Environmental Hazards

The health care professional needs to assess the cleanliness and level of repair of the home; the presence of pests; the adequacy of heat, water, electricity, gas, and ventilation; the functioning of kitchen and bathroom facilities; the adequacy of fire safety and equipment; and the presence of architectural barriers. Problems with any of these issues can result in serious difficulties for the elderly person as well as complicate the development of a care plan. The presence of an individual who has abused or threatened to abuse the elderly person is also an "environmental" problem that must be assessed like any other.

Severity and Intensity of Services Needed

After the health care professional has identified the major problems that are contributing to the presence of inadequate care, it is important to assess two additional dimensions of each problem—its severity and whether intervention must be continuous or intermittent. The severity of the problem helps to establish priorities for intervention. The intensity of services required provides a starting point for assessing the services that are currently available and need to be augmented in any care plan.

IDENTIFYING AVAILABLE RESOURCES

The issue at this point in the case management process is what resources are needed to resolve the inadequate care. Are they available from family, neighbors, friends, or other community resources, or are the care needs so great that acute or chronic institutionalization is required?

Even complicated medical, nursing, and mental health interventions can frequently be managed at home if the systems are in place to provide such care. The success of Hospice care testifies to the capacity of such systems to provide heroic services in very difficult circumstances. There are, however, some conditions that many community-based home care and nursing services find difficult to provide. Often, if the family or informal support system cannot provide these services, the only alternative to unsafe conditions and ongoing inadequate care is institutionalization. The need for 24-hour supervision because of impaired cognition cannot be met by most community agencies, nor can extremely intensive home services that require several different staff members on many separate occasions during a 24-hour period. This is due to limitations of both staff availability and the resources to pay for the services.

Before a care plan can be organized, it is also important for the health care professional to determine the stability of the sources of care, both formal and informal. There are limits to the expectations that can be placed on neighbors and friends for the ongoing care of an elderly person who is not related. The same is true of formal care systems, whose funding and staffing may be variable. Expectations of family members' participation are usually greater, but these people also may be limited by distance, job commitments, and financial constraints.

ASSESSING CARETAKER'S ROLE IN CREATING NEED

It is necessary to explore the possibility that the caretaker (if any) or other individual is contributing to care needs. This can occur through caretakers' active interference with the provision of services, through failure to provide care for which they are responsible, or by the creation of new needs for services by their actions. In addition to physical abuse that creates the need for protective and medical services, the failure to assure access to appropriate medical care can result in progressive disability and illness. While one assesses the possibility that the interventions of a caretaker, relative, or neighbor may be harmful rather than helpful, it is important not to discount the positive contributions that such individuals might make to the care of the elderly person, even though the sum of their interventions might be more harmful than helpful.

It is often not possible to ascertain directly from the elderly person whether they are experiencing abuse or neglect at the hands of a family member. Instead, one usually must infer this from a pattern of care needs that suggests that the caretaker is not providing adequate care or is actively creating care needs. If there is not a risk of imminent harm and intervention does not need to occur immediately, then there is time for the health care professional to address the unmet care needs of the elderly person while continuing to assess the situation. As long as care needs can be adequately addressed, it is not necessary to clarify immediately the caretaker's role in the development of inadequate care. If such a role becomes apparent in the course of developing a care plan, then the plan can be modified to account for the possibility of harmful behavior.

IDENTIFYING THE ELDER'S PRIORITIES

The final task of assessment is to identify the elderly person's priorities for intervention. Important as the preceding issues are, the client's priorities and willingness to accept an intervention plan are the keys to successful resolution of inadequate care. If the elder will not accept the care plan as proposed by the health care professional, then the preceding assessment will have been of little value. Identifying the client's priorities before a care plan is negotiated helps the health care professional to develop a plan that is more likely to be put into place. As part of a negotiating strategy, the health care provider can often gain the acceptance of an unwanted part of an intervention plan by the elderly person if the rest of the plan clearly addresses the person's priorities. There are no other ways to determine this except by asking the client.

While trying to determine the elder's priorities, it is important to emphasize that you are only trying to ascertain his or her wishes and are not trying to impose anything unwanted. This is accomplished by asking the elder explicity whether or not they value the resolution of a particular unmet care need. For example, in the case of an individual who is malnourished and manifests signs of poor hygiene, one could ask, "Is it important to you to be able to have meals on a regular basis?" "Would it be worthwhile to see if we can find a way to help keep yourself, your clothes, and your apartment clean?" In this way, one is able to help the elderly person identify the presence of unmet care needs. Having established their presence, the next step is to assist the elder in assigning a priority to meeting these care needs. It is at this point that the health care professional very often can help lead the elder through the process of decision-making and define priorities on the basis of the health care professional's perceived threat to the individual. In instances when the elder and the health care professional disagree on the priorities of resolving a particular unmet care need, it is in the best interests of maintaining and developing a long term care plan for the health care professional to work on the problems guided by the elder's priorities. The hope is that in the long run, by demonstrating the ability to work with the elderly person in resolving their most important (as defined by the elder) problems, the health care professional can then persuade the elderly person to deal with other issues.

SUMMARY

There are several dimensions to the process of assessment. There is a quantitative dimension measuring the extent of inadequate care and determining the degree of immediate risk or threat of imminent harm to the elderly person if the unmet care needs are not resolved. This dimension determines the pace of intervention. There is the qualitative dimension involving an assessment of the number, type, and severity of the unmet care needs and determining the potential extent of interventions. There is also an assessment of the resources available to the elderly person, including personal abilities, helpful family and neighbors, and professional caretakers. Knowing these factors helps to determine the range of intervention strategies that can be used. Finally, there is the presence or absence of evidence for abuse, which raises the issue of protective services. A comprehensive approach to assessment that includes each of these dimensions is the best method for effective patient care.

REFERENCES

Folstein, M. F., Folstein, S. E., & McHugh, P. R. (1975). Mini-Mental Method for Grading the Cognitive State of Patients for the Clinician. *Journal of Psychiatric Research, 12,* 189–198.

Kane, R. A., & Kane, R. L. (1981). *Assessing the Elderly: A Practical Guide to Measurement.* Lexington, MA: Lexington Books.

Lane v. Candura, 376 NE, 2nd, 1232, 1978.

6

Intervention

BASIC GUIDELINES

There are several lessons that we have learned by trial and error about intervention in abuse and neglect of the elderly. The first is that inadequate care frequently is of long duration and that rapid interventions are usually not necessary unless there is risk of imminent harm. The second is that most elderly persons value personal autonomy above personal safety and comfort, and, especially in the cases of those with families, most elderly persons would rather receive inadequate care living with their families than excellent care in an institution. The third is that assessment and intervention are best done by a multidisciplinary team because the issues of abuse, neglect, and inadequate care may involve medical, nursing, social service, legal, home care, mental health, and protective service professionals.

It is also important to understand that the goals of intervention are not established by the health care professional. The ultimate, ideal goal is the elimination of inadequate care. The goal that is more in accord with the actual limitations imposed by most elderly persons is to achieve a level of care that is acceptable to the client. This is not the same as eliminating inadequate care.

Unlike child abuse, where the goals of intervention are determined by the state and not the child or family, in abuse and neglect of the elderly, the client has the right to determine what outcome is most appropriate or acceptable. The goal of intervention, then, is to provide the elder with reasonable and acceptable options to a situation of abuse, neglect, or inadequate care. The analogy between child abuse and elder abuse ends here. As will be discussed in Chapter 8, the elderly person has the right to accept being abused. This greatly complicates the job of the health care professional.

The concept of "least restrictive alternative" is a principle that helps to guide the health care professional. The care plan in which the elderly has the greatest autonomy of action and that results in the level of resolution of inadequate care that is most acceptable to the elder is the least restrictive alternative. Only clients can define the alternatives that maximize their choices but involves the least disruption of their lifestyles. Home care services are less restrictive than institutional care; conservatorship is less restrictive than guardianship. Elderly persons will likely insist on the milder alternatives; if not, it is the health care professional's responsibility to consider them.

Since the health care professional cannot impose a care plan on the elderly client, such a plan must be negotiated. The professional may have to accept partial solutions to cases of inadequate care because the elder will not permit more extensive interventions. This is part of the challenge of caring for these individuals. The alternative—trying to impose a care plan on a competent elderly person—is, in itself, a denial of rights. The professional can only negotiate. The ability to negotiate skillfully, then, becomes an important professional attribute. Any strategies that increase one's ability to negotiate successfully should be used. These strategies include careful listening and attention to the elderly person's priorities and concerns.

THE ROLE OF THE HOSPITAL

Emergency unit teams play an important role in the detection of and intervention in inadequate care. Regardless of the elderly person's social situation, the response of the emergency room team should be to attempt to resolve the unmet needs and prevent further harm. The emergency room is frequently the patient's point of entry into the medical care system. The likelihood of successfully managing these cases over the long term is greatly affected by the outcome of the initial contact of the patient with the system. The emergency room team has a unique and essential role to play. To be successful requires the ability to correctly identify patients who are receiving inadequate care, assure their protection from further imminent harm, and facilitate the establishment of a long-term care plan. Failure to identify inadequate care or to successfully engage the patient in the resolution of the problem at the time of initial presentation may result in serious harm to the elderly person.

Correct emergency management of these patients requires an awareness of the manifestations of abuse and neglect; knowledge of appropriate strategies of intervention given the context of the inadequate care; and backup by a multidisciplinary team. A satisfactory resolution is also facilitated by focusing on the identification and resolution of the care needs of elderly people, rather than on the acts or omissions of their caretakers. This approach is less threatening to both clients and caretakers, and the emphasis on concrete problems and their solutions helps to establish a supportive relationship with the elders. Confrontational or accusatory actions on the part of the emergency room staff may increase the elders' reluctance to acknowledge the problem and result in their refusal to permit assessment or intervention. Fear of nursing home placement, retaliation by family members, or confinement may make them reluctant to discuss the issue, regardless of a tactful and sensitive approach by the emergency room staff.

The urgency with which supportive and/or protective services need to be provided is determined by the extent of the risk of imminent harm. When the risk is great, hospital admission is usually warranted. Admission is most frequently acceptable to both the elderly person and the family member when it is justified in terms of treatment for a specific problem rather than as protection from further abuse or neglect. The emergency room staff should facilitate rather than impede the admission of such cases, as hospitalization has several advantages over trying to set up an elaborate home care plan during a brief emergency room visit. Access to the elderly person for assessment and intervention may not be possible once the elderly person goes home. Hospitalization is a socially acceptable way to separate a stressed or abusive caretaker from the elder. It is usually possible to establish a relationship between the caretaker and a health care professional while the stressed caretaker's need for respite is being met. Such relationships are important for the long-term management of these cases. Hospitalization also provides adequate time to define the actual care needs of the elder and to arrange for services to meet them. The time and opportunity to perform an adequate assessment and to negotiate interventions are extremely important; hospitalization permits the involvement of a multidisciplinary team to accomplish this.

Because of the elder's right to refuse services, we must frequently accept solutions that we consider to be inadequate. It is therefore important to keep negotiations with the elderly person flexible and to concentrate on maintaining access and follow-up. This is so that additions to the care plan can be made over time as the health care team gains the elder's trust.

If hospitalization appears warranted because of the risk of imminent harm but is not acceptable to the elderly person, then the appropriate response is to initiate an assessment of how the individual's activities of daily living are accomplished (or not) and who provides the necessary assistance. Although home care may appear to be inadequate to prevent further abuse or neglect, it must be pursued if it is the only intervention permitted by the client.

THE PROCESS OF INTERVENTION

Figure 6-1 presents an overview of the process of intervention. It begins during the process of assessment, imme-

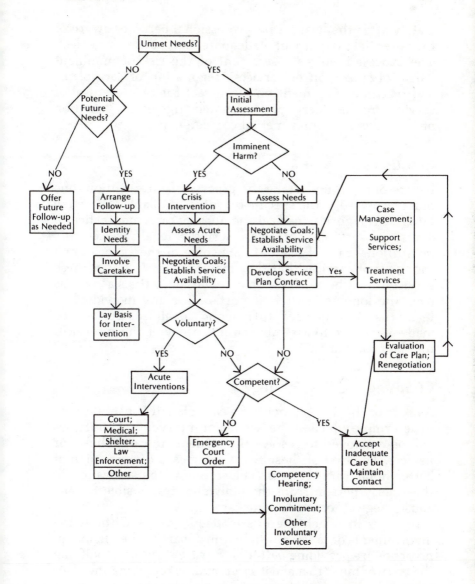

FIGURE 6-1 Overview of the process of intervention

diately after the health care professional becomes aware of the potential existence of inadequate care, abuse, or neglect. The process involves assessment of the risk of imminent harm, organization of services, negotiation of care plans, and reaching agreement on a contract for care. Refusal of services by the elderly person should trigger an evaluation of the elderly person's mental competency.

Resources

Before one can undertake the process of intervention, one must be aware of the specific resources available. These fall into five categories: medical and nursing care, mental health and social services, home care services, legal services, and institutional care. Table 6-1 lists some of the agencies and the types of services that they may provide. Many of these services must be available on an emergency basis as well as over the long term. It is important for any individual or team that is organized to respond to abuse, neglect, or inadequate care to assemble an inventory of these services for their local area.

Choosing the Best Strategy

As part of the development of a care plan, it is useful to try to determine which of the two major intervention strategies will be employed to resolve the inadequate care, abuse, or neglect. The first of these two strategies is the provision of better home care services. The second is the separation of the elderly person from the individual responsible for the abuse, neglect, or inadequate care.

In cases in which there is inadequate care without the involvement of a responsible third party, the main approaches are providing better home care services, modifying the environment to make it safer, and/or removing the elder from the unsafe environment because adequate home care services are not available. Cases where the risk of imminent harm is from untreated medical problems, cognitive impairment, or lack of personal care services fall into this category, and interventions should concentrate on resolving these unmet care needs.

In contrast, in cases where the risk of imminent harm is from the presence of an individual who has harmed or is threatening to harm the elder, separation of the elder and the abuser must be considered. In these situations the abuser may in fact be creating needs for care that were nonexistent before. Separation then provides complete resolution of the unmet care needs. However, these cases are frequently complicated when the abuser has a significant caretaking role in addition to any other negative aspects of his or her behavior. In these situations it is essential to replace the caretaking services provided by the abuser prior to completing the strategy to separate the abuser and the elderly person.

Figure 6–2 describes the process of developing a care plan when the major issue confronting the health care professional is whether or not the elderly person is dependent on others to meet his or her current care needs. Figure 6–3 describes the issues that must be clarified before an elderly person can be separated from an abuser. The selection of services and the problems that must be resolved are different in these different types of cases, and there are areas where the two processes overlap. Before the separation strategy is employed, one major consideration must be to ensure that any care needs the abuser may have been supplying can be replicated in the care plan in a minimally restrictive way. If this is not possible, then separation from the abuser might not be acceptable to the elder, especially if the alternative is institutional care.

It is becoming apparent from our discussion that the complexity of these situations asks us to break them down into manageable pieces, by attempting to categorize the cases in some way. It has not been demonstrated to be particularly useful to separate cases of inadequate care on the basis of the type of abuse or neglect (such as active or passive neglect, financial exploitation, denial of rights, or

TABLE 6-1 Agencies and Services Available for Abuse, Neglect, and Inadequate Care

Department of Social Services:
  Financial assistance
  Homemaker services
  Counseling
  Foster care and residential treatment
  Payment for emergency shelter; security deposits for apartments
  Transportation
Mental Health Agencies:
  Crisis counseling
  Family outreach
  Assessment for psychiatric care/commitment
  Individual, marital, family, and group psychotherapy
  Partial hospitalization (therapeutic daycare)
Hospitals:
  Alcohol or drug detoxification
  In-patient psychiatric treatment
  Emergency medical care
  Inpatient medical treatment
Public Health Agencies; Private Physicians:
  Dental care
  Home health aide service
  Outpatient medical care
Employment Agencies & Services:
  Career counseling
  Job training and placement
  Vocational rehabilitation
  Adult education for other family members
Alcohol/Drug Treatment Agencies:
  Residential treatment
  Home or outpatient counseling
  Service for other family members
Nursing Homes:
  Custodial care
  Daycare
  Respite care
  Self-help groups (AA, Al-Anon)
Volunteer Agencies:
  Emergency food, clothing, and shelter
  Transportation (emergency or support)

TABLE 6–1 (*Continued*)

Support groups
Friendly visitor programs
Recreation
Socialization
Hotlines
Women's advocacy and counseling groups
Housing Services:
Emergency shelter/crisis housing
Group home or adult foster home setting
Assistance with securing affordable, permanent housing
Law Enforcement Agency:
Crisis intervention
Arrest of abuser
Magistrate:
Warrant for arrest
Civil Courts:
Competency hearings
Psychiatric commitment
Orders for medical and/or psychiatric care
Hearings for assault, separation
Protective orders (injunctions and restraining orders; peace bond; torts; court conciliation/mediation)
Criminal Courts:
Arrest warrant
Arraignment
Preliminary hearing
Trial for assault
Imprisonment
Fine
Probation
Legal Services:
Consultation regarding legal rights
Advice regarding filing arrest warrants and petitioning the court for separation
Representation in court
Advocacy with Welfare and other agencies

Source: Adapted from U.S. Department of Health and Human Services. *Family Violence: Intervention Strategies.* DHHS Pub. No. (OHDS) 80-30258. 1980, pp. 52–54. Washington, DC: U.S. Government Printing Office.

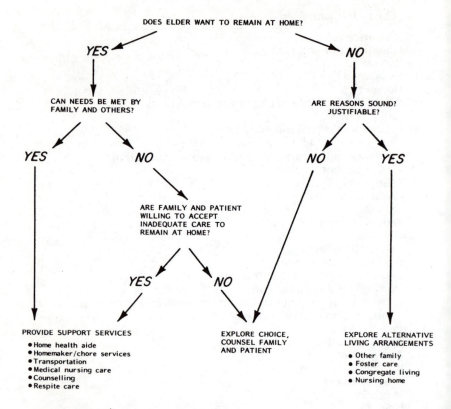

FIGURE 6–2 Decision flow chart for abuse or neglect of elderly person dependent on others for care.

Source: T. A. O'Malley, D. E. Everitt, H. C. O'Malley, & E. W. Campion. Identifying and Preventing Family-Mediated Abuse and Neglect of Elderly Persons. *Annals of Internal Medicine, 98*(6), 1983, 998–1005, Figure 1. Reprinted with permission.

verbal abuse), nor on the basis of the elderly person's presentation to the care system (signs of dehydration, trauma, cognitive impairment, or poor hygiene). However, there are some parameters that can be used to separate cases in ways that help guide intervention. Some of these processes are outlined in Figures 6–2 and 6–3. In particular, it is possible to identify subgroups of elderly persons who live at home with family and are receiving inadequate care. They are categorized on the basis of (1) their care needs and (2) the significance of the caretaking role of the individual felt to be responsible for the inadequate care. These two items have practical importance in choosing appropriate interventions. As will be discussed later in the chapter, they also have prognostic significance for outcome.

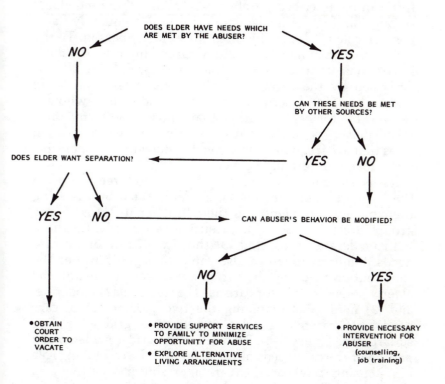

FIGURE 6–3 Decision flow chart for abuse or neglect of elderly person by a pathologic abuser.

Source: T. A. O'Malley, D. E. Everitt, H. C. O'Malley, & E. W. Campion. Identifying and Preventing Family-Mediated Abuse and Neglect of Elderly Persons. *Annals of Internal Medicine, 98*(6), 1983, 998–1005, Figure 2. Reprinted with permission.

Thus, it is possible to categorize elders on the basis of their care needs and the significance of the caretaking role of the individual felt to be responsible for the inadequate care. This individual can be described as a "caretaker-abuser." The term is meant to be a shorthand description of those individuals who are responsible for abuse, neglect, or other forms of inadequate care. Except in those instances where the individual has no caretaking responsibilities and therefore can be described purely as an "abuser," the individual responsible for the inadequate care quite frequently has a positive role to play in the care of the elderly person. To the extent that they have a beneficial caretaking role, the duality of their contribution to the elder's well-being is best described by the term "caretaker-abuser." Also included under the same description are those individuals who are responsible for neglect rather than abuse. The term "caretaker-abuser" is only meant to describe the two conflicting roles that are frequently assumed by individuals responsible for inadequate care of the elderly.

It is possible to divide elderly persons into three groups on the basis of their care needs, as determined by assessing their medical problems and their functional status. These groups are (1) those with extensive care needs, (2) those with moderate needs, and (3) those with few or no care needs. Similarly, one can also rank the significance of the contribution made by the caretaker-abuser in meeting the elderly person's need for care as (1) extensive, (2) moderate, and (3) minimal. Combining the two parameters of care needs and caretaking roles results in a grid with nine squares (see Figure 6-4). Each cell in the grid is made up of a pairing of the care needs of the elder and the caretaking role (*not* abusing role) of the caretaker-abuser. As the grid shows, those situations in which the caretaking role of the caretaker-abuser is greater than the care needs of the elder represent adequate care. Those situations in which the care needs of the elder exceed the caretaking role of the caretaker-abuser represent inadequate care. Those situations in which the care needs and the caretaking role appear to be

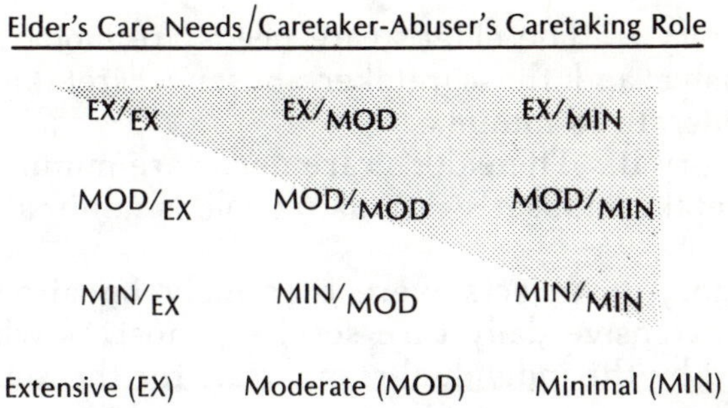

Elder's Care Needs/Caretaker-Abuser's Caretaking Role

EX/EX	EX/MOD	EX/MIN
MOD/EX	MOD/MOD	MOD/MIN
MIN/EX	MIN/MOD	MIN/MIN

Extensive (EX)   Moderate (MOD)   Minimal (MIN)

FIGURE 6–4 Variations in the relationship between elder's needs and care received leading to potential inadequate care (shaded area).

roughly equal represent cases in which the care may be adequate or inadequate. The three cells on the diagonal slant from upper left to lower right and the three cells in the upper righthand corner of the grid represent situations of inadequate care. They can be combined into three separate categories based on the extent of the caretaking needs and the extent of the caretaking role. At the two extremes are those cases falling into the upper lefthand corner of the grid and the lower righthand corner, where the caretaking needs of the elderly person are either very extensive and matched by an extensive caretaking role, or minimal matched by a minimal caretaking role. A middle category includes those cases in the upper righthand corner of the grid in which the caretaking needs of the elderly person are significantly greater than the caretaking role and the caretaking role of the caretaker-abuser. It is in this disparity that abuse, neglect, and inadequate care occur.

We conducted a study of cases of inadequate care based on these categories to classify the cases (O'Malley et al., 1984). The three categories of inadequate care that we worked with were as follows:

Category I: The elder's care needs are extensive and the caretaker-abuser's caretaking role is extensive.

Category II: The elder's care needs are moderate to extensive and the caretaker-abuser's caretaking role is moderate to minimal.

Category III: The elder's care needs are minimal and the caretaker-abuser's caretaking role is minimal.

Category I subjects were extremely impaired and required extensive daily care services, most of which were provided by the individual responsible for the abuse or neglect. The resulting manifestations of inadequate care were predominantly those of neglect, such as unmet medical needs, worsening decubiti, malnutrition, and dehydration. Episodes of verbal or physical abuse were rare. In our experience, all of these individuals required hospitalization, and most cases were resolved by placement in chronic-care facilities that could adequately meet the elderly person's needs for daily care. Those not requiring placement were managed by adding extensive home care services to assist the existing caretaker. The cases were generally of short duration (several months) and did not involve battering or psychological abuse. The resulting inadequate care appeared to be due to a lack of ability or training on the part of the caretaker. The caretaker-abuser was most often a spouse. In this situation, the caretaker-abuser includes those individuals who neglect, for whatever reason, care needs of the elderly person. This is not meant to imply that the cases in this category represent abuse. By and large they are cases of neglect rather than abuse.

Category II subjects were found to be moderately to extremely impaired individuals who were socially isolated and required moderate to extensive personal care services on a daily basis. Most of these care services were either not provided or were provided only intermittently by the individual responsible for the elderly person's care. In the face of very significant care needs, the caretaker's response was inadequate either in quantity, range, or frequency, similar to the actions of caretakers in Category I. However, the cases in Category II included battering, psychological abuse, and misuse of resources, in addition to unmet medical needs, as in Category I. The presence of these other manifestations of abuse and inadequate care in Category II clearly distinguishes these cases from those in Category I. The characteristics of the caretaker-abuser, the duration of the inadequate care, and the interventions used to resolve these cases were also different than those in Category I.

Hospitalization was often used as a means to separate elderly victims from their caretaker-abusers, as well as to treat significant medical problems. The caretaker-abuser was most often an offspring or sibling and frequently had mental health problems or abused alcohol. Episodes of abuse and neglect occurred over a period of months to years, and most of these cases remained incompletely resolved, despite attempts at intervention, because of resistance by the victims and the caretaker-abusers. Often, an abuser realized financial gain from keeping his or her dependent parent at home. These were the most difficult cases to resolve because frequently the elderly person did not want to disrupt the relationship with his or her child, despite the abuse and neglect. Resolution, when it occurred, usually was achieved only by separation through nursing home placement.

Subjects in Category III were independent and required little or no assistance with activities of daily living. The manifestations of inadequate care in these cases were primarily those of abuse and included battering, anxiety, fear, and depression. There was also significant misuse of resources such as extortion of funds by violence or threat of violence. In these cases there was no caretaking role for the individual responsible for the abuse to assume; therefore, the term "abuser" appears to be more appropriate in this instance than the term "caretaker-abuser." Although the caretaking role of these individuals was minimal, they frequently created serious requirements for protective services and inflicted much injury on these elderly individuals. The abuser was most often a grandchild of the subject. Drug abuse by the abuser was frequently cited as a cause. The episodes of abuse frequently extended over many years but were nearly always resolved through interventions that either separated the elderly person from the abuser or significantly modified the abuser's behavior.

Table 6–2 summarizes the interventions that were used in these three categories of cases.

A TEAM APPROACH TO INTERVENTION

Selection of a particular intervention plan and its successful negotiation require a multidisciplinary approach. All cases require long-term monitoring, frequent evaluation at home, and adjustment of support services to match increasing care needs. A team approach involving the physician, home care nurse, home care services coordinator, and social service worker is most effective.

Beth Israel Hospital Elder Assessment Team

The Beth Israel Hospital Elder Assessment Team in Boston is an example of the type of organization required to address issues of abuse, neglect, and inadequate care. This group has been functioning since 1981 as a multidisciplinary team which has, as its central task, the assessment of all referred cases of suspected abuse and neglect within the hospital system (Carr et al., 1986). The team is composed of nurses, physicians, and social workers who evaluate re-

TABLE 6–2 Interventions Used in Three Categories

Category	Types of Intervention
I	1, 2
II	1, 2, 3, 4
III	3, 4

Key: 1 = homecare services; 2 = nursing home, chronic care; 3 = separation, new caretaker; 4 = legal sanctions.

ferred cases and make recommendations to the hospital administration as to whether, in the clinical judgment of the team, a report should be made to the appropriate state agency. The team also provides consultation regarding appropriate plans of care for abused or neglected elders, which might include obtaining restraining orders for abusers, increased home health care supports, or long-term care placement.

Each plan of care is carefully individualized in order to take into account the unique circumstances of each case. In no situation is a plan of care forced upon an elder. The team is there to provide support to the primary caregivers in the hospital, who are struggling with difficult clinical and ethical issues that often arise in elder abuse and neglect cases. Modeled after similar abuse intervention teams (Bittner & Newberger, 1981), the team is seen as a group of experts who can provide an in-depth assessment when cases of suspected abuse or neglect arise. This is extremely helpful for busy clinicians who have a "feeling" that something may not be right and yet do not feel they have the knowledge base to determine if abuse or neglect has occurred.

The Elder Assessment Team (EAT) reviews the patient's recent and past medical records, interviews the patient and family members when possible, examines the patient, and talks directly to care providers. The team then makes a recommendation to the hospital administration as to whether it feels a state report is necessary. The hospital administrator is the person who calls in the report, however, as members of the team feel strongly that it is important to maintain a clinical focus. Any member of the hospital staff may choose to circumvent the EAT process and make a formal report at any time.

Since it was organized, the EAT has served in a consultative manner for abuse or neglect cases and as an in-service educational resource at the Beth Israel Hospital. Team members also have frequently been called upon to provide educational programs at local, state, and national meetings. Some members also serve on policy boards that are developing rules and regulations for defining and describing elder abuse and neglect.

In the event that a patient who is not likely to be admitted is referred to the team from the emergency unit, assessment must be immediate. In cases where the patient is going to be admitted to the hospital, the team has more time to perform an assessment. The team is available during regular working hours on the weekdays. On weekends and off-shifts, the clinical advisors in nursing, who are available in-house by page, serve as the on-site administrators responsible for assessing and triaging the patient appropriately. All clinical advisors have received special training on the topic of elder abuse and are familiar with hospital policy for intervention.

Forming Your Own Elder Abuse Team

Elder abuse teams provide a mechanism for discussion, education, and clinical evaluation of suspected elder abuse cases in a consistent and dependable manner. Composition of such teams will vary from organization to organization; depending on the purpose of the organization and its dominant employee group. For example, hospital-based teams will usually consist of physicians, nurses, social workers, and relevant therapists, while social service agency teams will likely consist of social workers and caseworkers from varying backgrounds. The key element is interest and commitment to the development of a structure for reviewing suspected elder abuse cases in a way that is feasible, given organizational time constraints and funding issues.

Few institutions or agencies will be willing to fund a new position for elder abuse work; however, most will agree to incorporate such work into an existing position. Some agencies will need to rely heavily on existing state agency programs for assessment and care planning, while others will need only minimal direction. Hospitals or Visiting Nurses' Associations with geriatricians or nurse specialists in geriatrics can provide extremely useful expertise for use in avoid-

ing overreporting and mislabeling common geriatric problems as abuse.

Teams should plan to meet on a regular basis to review
cases, delineate agency policies, and plan in-service education. It is important to keep accurate minutes of such meetings in order to provide records of group decisions. An
agency administrator should be involved either as a team
member or consultant to the group, in order to insure that
all processes and decisions are congruent with the agency
policies.

As soon as a team or advisory group has been named, its
members will need to consider their own educational needs
as well as the projected needs of agency staff. A regular
program of elder abuse seminars conducted by knowledgeable professionals will probably by the most efficient way to
disseminate information. For individuals who work on a
part-time or off-shift basis, self-paced teaching modules
that include key journal articles and assessment instruments can be provided. Follow-up can be conducted by telephone discussion or through mail correspondence. A contact person should be identified for any questions related to
such material. Films that discuss elder abuse may also be
helpful and can be ordered through local libraries or state
agencies. Finally, it is especially helpful to provide written
agency guidelines for elder abuse reporting criteria so that
individuals have a ready reference. *Elder Abuse Report*, published by the University of Massachusetts Center on Aging,
is a quarterly newsletter that provides a forum for dissemi-
nating information on the subject.

Once an organization initiates the development of an
elder abuse screening and reporting process, it is important
that community agencies be informed that such a program
is under way. There is a great deal of suspicion and mistrust
surrounding the issue of elder abuse assessment. Local nursing homes, hospitals, and social service agencies may feel
threatened and regard such a project as unwarranted peer
review of existing care. In the case of the elderly, it is not
unlikely that three or four agencies are involved in provid-

ing care on a regular basis. If an elderly person from a nursing home presents in an emergency unit and is assessed for possible abuse or neglect, careful measures need to be taken to alert that nursing home that such an assessment is being conducted. Information should be conveyed in a non-accusatory manner, with the purpose of such communication being that of data gathering. Frequently, such suspected cases can be readily explained, as in the following:

> An elderly woman presented in the emergency unit from a local nursing home with multiple upper-body bruises and no documentation of their etiology. The patient was cognitively impaired and unable to give an account of the incident. Suspecting abuse, the staff nurse called the nursing home to determine the source of the bruising. The nursing home physician explained that the patient had episodes of agitation that warranted the use of restraints. Due to the patient's poor nutritional status, however, bruises occurred easily when she pulled on the restraints, even though extra padding had been provided.

This case illustrates the point that what may appear to be an abuse event may actually be the result of a health problem. Reynolds and Stanton (1983) makes this same point when they state the following:

> Many families take the responsibility of caring for their elderly relatives who may be severely physically impaired. They may be readmitted to the hospital in what appears to be a sad state of neglect. They may have decubitus ulcers, and their nutritional state may be poor. Abuse may be suspected; but, in reality, these families were not given sufficient education to care for their elderly relatives, and needed services were not made available to them. It is difficult for a senile 86-year-old man to care properly for his physically impaired 84-year-old wife. But, many patients leave emergency departments and hospital units with inadequate patient education and a haphazard assessment of their needs. [p. 400]

The importance of interagency communication can readily be discerned. Each agency should identify a liaison mechanism for following elderly persons as they pass through the various levels of health care. Such community networks enhance the quality of health care for the elderly and eliminate suspicion and mistrust among agencies.

It is important to discuss whether "protective service admissions" are still feasible under the current reimbursement system. With the initiation of DRGs (Diagnostic Related Groupings), hospitals are reimbursed prospectively on the basis of the admitting diagnosis. "Need for protective service" is not a recognized DRG category, and reimbursement to the hospital for such admissions is problematic. However, it is extremely important for health care professionals who are charged with the responsibility of performing elder abuse assessments to discuss this issue with relevant hospital administrators so that everyone involved is clear about the policy of the institution. In some states, protective services such as emergency housing are available through the appropriate state agencies. In other states, such services may not be available and hospitals may be put in the position of considering whether or not an elder, who does not necessarily need a medical admission, needs a protective service admission. It has been our experience that a policy for providing a protective service admission is an important one. When no alternative is available, the elderly person who may be a victim of abuse or neglect requires a safe environment and the hospital is in a position to provide such an environment. In the past five years, no more than two protective service admissions per year have been documented at the Beth Israel Hospital in Boston as resulting from a concern regarding possible elder abuse or neglect.

In addition to intervening in existing cases, inadequate care is an important task of any assessment team. In fact, the team has a responsibility to help shift the emphasis of intervention toward prevention. This can be done in several ways. First, the team should have a role in teaching assessment techniques to other health care professionals so that a "geriatric sensitivity" is developed. This approach should emphasize the consideration of the functional status and health care needs of all elderly persons who are encountered in the system. If other health care providers could be persuaded to be sensitive to the difficulties imposed by functional limitations on the daily routine of the elderly person, fewer elderly persons would be discharged prematurely from the hospital or prescribed treatments that are unrealistic because of the lack of supportive services.

Second, careful discharge planning is essential. For patients going home, it is important to assess the need for and availability of supportive services prior to discharge. Caretakers must be adequately trained and supported. The team must be able to anticipate potential problems and develop alternative care plans to resolve them. For elderly persons who are being transferred to a long-term-care facility, the referring hospital has the responsibility of assuring that the facility provides acceptable care. Hospitals unwittingly contribute to the inadequate care of the elderly by referring patients to long-term-care facilities that have poor records of patient care. Unfortunately, the financial pressures on hospitals to discharge patients quickly can contribute to the development of inadequate care. It is the responsibility of the medical, nursing, and social service staffs to see that the well-being of the patient comes before the financial interests of the institution.

FOLLOW-UP

Follow-up can be one of the most difficult aspects of an elder abuse case for the health care professional. Once an emergent situation has been resolved, the tendency is to relax the intensity of the vigilance previously given to the situation. Whereas it may be appropriate in some cases to do so, it is important to develop a system in which the elderly person can be monitored over time to ensure his or her safety. Situations may change over time and as the elderly person advances in age, inadequate care may increase. Frequent contact between the elderly person and a health care professional is the basis for continuing surveillance of the elderly person.

There are many ways to assure regular contact. Periodic physical examinations for chronic health problems are a good opportunity for evaluating the quality of the elderly person's current living situation and determining if there is a notable increase in actual or potential unmet needs. In cases that involve elderly persons with cognitive impairments or those who are living with individuals who have a documented psychiatric disorder or mental retardation, it is important to consider the use of periodic home visits in addition to office visits to ensure elders' safety.

Regular visits by home care nurses are an effective means to assure follow-up of those elderly persons needing ongoing medical care. However, as a practical point, it may be difficult to obtain reimbursement for these visits unless there are resources earmarked for protective services or there are unstable medical conditions that qualify the visit for payment by a third party insurer. In many cases, however, this is not possible and home care agencies must provide this service without reimbursement. This is a major barrier for providing adequate care to these elderly persons.

Home visits by social service–mental health workers are also useful means for assuring follow-up as well as for providing guidance for crisis resolution and prevention. They can also provide ongoing support for elderly persons who are depressed and socially isolated. Unfortunately, fiscal constraints are even greater on social service–mental health visits than they are on "medical" services. Unless specific resources are allocated to pay for these services they are often impossible to continue for any significant length of time.

The advantage of having home visits performed by skilled medical or mental health personnel is that they are trained to identify and react to potential problems. This capability cannot be substituted for by using other, less extensively trained individuals such as homemakers, home health aides, or "friendly visitors." However, it is clear from many reports that the regular presence of almost any outside visitor in the home is sufficient to decrease significantly the frequency and extent of abuse and neglect. This may be due to its effect on lessening the elderly person's social isolation as well as increasing the likelihood of adverse consequences on the perpetrator.

Whether the home visits are performed by a physician, nurse, social worker, or home health aide, home monitoring is an essential and effective means of assuring follow-up. In the course of negotiating with a client or family about intervention, it is important to set the stage for home visits to assure long-term monitoring.

There can be great variability among cases in terms of how quickly they are resolved, how completely they are resolved, and how stable they remain over time. Because it may not be possible to predict at the outset what will happen with any individual case, long-term monitoring becomes essential to assure that problems that have been resolved remain resolved; and problems that have not been resolved remain under attention. However, despite the difficulty in predicting the outcome of any one case, it is possible to identify categories of cases that share similar outcomes.

In Table 6–2 we described categories of cases of abuse and neglect that were derived from the extent of the care needs of the elderly persons and the extent of individual caretaking roles. Category I cases involved elderly persons with extensive care needs who were inadequately cared for despite intensive efforts on the part of their caretakers. Category II cases involved elderly persons with extensive care needs that were responded to infrequently, inconsistently, and inadequately. Those individuals who were responsible for meeting the care needs of the elderly person often were responsible for creating some of those care needs. Category

TABLE 6-3

Category	Types of Intervention	Outcome (O'Malley et al., 1984)
I	1, 2	Good
II	1, 2, 3, 4	Poor
III	3, 4	Good

Key: 1 = homecare services; 2 = nursing home, chronic care; 3 = separation, new caretaker; 4 = legal sanctions.

III cases involved elderly persons who had no care needs except for the need for protective services created by the actions of a relative who had no caretaking role. In general, cases in each of these categories required different interventions and had different outcomes.

Table 6-3 summarizes the interventions used with cases in each of these three categories. A "good" outcome is the resolution of inadequate care and the development of a system of monitoring and services that assure that inadequate care will not recur. A "poor" outcome is the failure to resolve significant unmet needs for any reason or the inability to develop a system for ongoing monitoring in those cases in which unmet needs were only partially resolved.

Category I cases all required more intensive levels of services. But once appropriate services were provided, inadequate care ceased. There were no issues of physical abuse, financial exploitation, or denial of rights. Ongoing monitoring was essential in order to assure that the elderly person's needs for medical care and assistance with activities of daily living continued to be met by the current plan. The major difficulty encountered in managing these cases was confronting the need for institutionalized care when care needs exceeded the capacity of the caretaker and system to provide services at home.

Category II cases had a uniformly poor outcome despite using all interventions possible. The inadequate or ambivalent responses of caretakers to established care needs or their participation in creating needs made them uncertain partners at best in resolving inadequate care. Often, financial exploitation was the driving force in these cases and proved to be difficult to change because the elderly person's assets were the only resources available to support the rest of the family. These cases were the most difficult to gain access to, the most difficult to negotiate interventions with, and the most difficult with which to establish any long-term monitoring.

Despite all of these difficulties, it is important for the health care professional to make whatever small gains are possible in reducing the burden of unmet care needs. Often in these cases one must accept inadequate care that would not be tolerated in another case, only because it is an improvement, however slight, over what preceded it. Because the intervention options permitted by the elderly person are so limited, it is important to concentrate on maintaining access rather than promoting other types of intervention. Over time, it may be possible to negotiate more extensive interventions, but that is only possible if access can be maintained.

Category III cases involved abusive or coercive acts by a relative against an otherwise independent elderly person who had no unmet ongoing care needs. The main difficulty in these cases was to convince the elderly person that there are effective ways to prevent this from happening and to overcome their reluctance to involve outsiders in a "family problem." Because there was no need to construct an elaborate care plan or involve the relative in that plan, these cases were the easiest to resolve. The difficulty rested with engaging the elderly person rather than developing a care plan. Ongoing monitoring of these cases could usually be done by telephone or by enlisting friends and neighbors to report any recurrence.

Institutionalized elderly persons represent another group whose follow-up must be monitored closely. This is especially true if they are returned to the same institution in which the inadequate care occurred. It is essential that steps are taken within the institution to prevent any recurrence. This may include staff transfer or dismissal, staff education, or changes in patient care review. It is also essential that there is an outside group that also monitors the care of the elderly person. This could be the state or regional agency that is responsible for certifying the adequacy of all nursing homes or it could be the elder abuse team that was responsible for managing the patient while hospitalized.

Good patient care probably requires that elderly persons not be returned to the original facility, but rather transferred to a new long-term care facility. Part of the responsibility of the intervention team is to identify substandard long-term care facilities, to avoid making referrals to them, and to report cases of inadequate care to the appropriate licensing boards.

Abuse and neglect of elderly persons in nursing homes is probably seriously underreported. The more nursing homes are open to scrutiny by families, regulatory agencies, and outside visitors, the less likely it is that abuse and neglect will occur. Well-trained senior staff and the commitment of management to assuring swift resolution of suspected abuse or neglect of patients is essential.

The development of standards of care for commonly encountered problems in nursing homes could be of significant help in eliminating abuse and neglect if they were applied to all long-term care facilities. The care of patients with incontinence, malnutrition, decubiti, and those requiring restraints (chemical and physical) could be improved by the implementation of standards of care. This might also help nursing home staffs develop approaches to the patient that make inadequate care less likely. When pride in the standard of care is not enough to prevent inadequate care of institutionalized elderly persons, then severe penalties for both the responsible staff member and institution need to be invoked.

REFERENCES

Bittner, S., & Newburger, E. (1981). Pediatric Understanding of Abuse and Neglect. *Pediatrics in Review, 2*(1), 197–208.

Carr, K., Dix, G., Fulmer, T., Kavesh, W., Kravitz, L., Matlaw, J., Mayer, J., Minaker, K., Shapiro, M., Street, S., Wetle, T., & Zarle, N. (1986). An Elder Abuse Assessment Team in an Acute Hospital Setting. *The Gerontologist, 26*(2), 115–118.

O'Malley, T. A., Everitt, P. E., O'Malley, H. C., & Campion, E. W. (1983). Identifying and preventing family-mediated abuse and neglect of elderly persons. *Annals of Internal Medicine, 98*(6, Part 1), 998–1005.

O'Malley, T. A., O'Malley, H. C., Everitt, D. E., & Sarson, D. (1984). Catagories of family-mediated abuse and neglect of elderly persons. *Journal of the American Geriatrics Society, 32*(5), 362–369.

Reynolds, E., & Stanton, S. (1983). Elderly Abuse in a Hospital: A Nursing Perspective. In J. Kosberg (Ed.), *Abuse and Maltreatment of the Elderly: Causes and Interventions* (pp. 391–403). Boston: PSG Publishing.

7

Elder Abuse Reporting Laws and Decisions to Report

A comprehensive history of all types of abuse legislation as well as information about the current status of federal legislation to prevent and resolve the national problem of elder abuse is given in Oakar and Miller (1983). According to them, child abuse was the first form of family violence to be addressed by national organizations when, in 1874, the case of Mary Ellen Wilson was pleaded by, of all people, the American Society for the Prevention of Cruelty to Animals (ASPCA). It seems shocking that the ASPCA was founded before any such organization existed for humans, but that was the case. As a result of this landmark case, Eldridge T. Gerry founded the New York Society for the Prevention of Cruelty to Children in December 1874. Soon after, the State of New York enacted the country's first child abuse law, and by 1922 there were 56 societies for the prevention of cruelty to children.

It was not until the early 1960s that research was published on the topic of child abuse in medical journals. With such documentation, governmental action was swift; by 1966, 49 states had enacted legislation mandating reporting of any suspected cases of child abuse by health care providers. On January 31, 1974, the Child Abuse Prevention and Treatment Act (P.L. 93–247) was enacted to provide federal monies for the prevention and treatment of child abuse. Through these measures, which drew attention to the horrors of child abuse, issues of family violence emerged indicating that it was not only children who were victims of domestic violence. During the 1970s there was much writing and research regarding battered women. Finally, in the 1980s, has come a time for evaluation of the nature and scope of elder abuse.

The first congressional hearing that specifically addressed abuse of the elderly was held on June 23, 1979, by the House Select Committee on Aging, in Boston, Massachusetts (U.S. House, 1979). A second hearing followed on April 21, 1980, in New York City, held by the Subcommittee on Human Services of the House Select Committee on Aging, followed by a comparable hearing in Union, New Jersey one week later (U.S. House of Representatives, 1980). Through these and similar hearings, stories of abuse and neglect were unveiled to a shocked legislature and public, stories that clearly documented the phenomenon of elder abuse and the urgent need for prevention programs, better research, and public education.

ELDER ABUSE LEGISLATION

To date, there is no federal legislation related to elder abuse. While bills have been introduced, they have yet to pass, probably due to their exorbitant pricetags. The cost of enforcing these measures was estimated by the Congressional Budget Office as $4.5 million in 1982, increasing to $12.5 million by 1986. While federal legislation is pending, the ways in which individual states address programatic issues and budgetary allowances vary widely.

There are now 30 states that have passed mandatory reporting laws for elder abuse (Cohen, 1984). These laws encompass a wide range of definitions, and few states have good documentation of the actual physical, emotional, or material abuse situations that allegedly have occurred. The variety of definitions as well as the differences in the evaluation process make it impossible to compare data from one state to another. One study (Salend, Kane, Satz, & Pynoos, 1984) compared 16 state elderly abuse reporting statutes and analyzed the implementation process. They found that key terms such as *abuse*, *neglect*, and *exploitation* were unstandardized and vague. "For example," they stated, "the definition of 'abuse' in one statute was equivalent to the definition of 'neglect' in another. Exploitation, the phenomenon most uniformly defined in the statutes, commonly meant improper use of another's assets for one's own profit" (p. 62).

These laws do perform an important function, however, of heightening awareness regarding the problem of elder abuse. They also increase health care provider sensitivity in that failure to report suspected elder abuse is usually prosecutable, and professionals who fail to report are usually subject to some penalty, such as fines or revocation of professional license.

In those states that do not have specific elder abuse reporting laws, such abuse is legally covered under other protective service legislation that may encompass a wider age range (i.e., 18 years of age or older). Thobaben and Anderson (1985) have summarized such legislation for all 50 states and note that, as of February 1985, only nine states have no laws that encompass elder abuse. Those states are Indiana, Kansas, Maryland, Mississippi, North Dakota, New York, New Jersey, Pennsylvania, and South Dakota. Each state designates appropriate agencies to accept reports for elder abuse and provide guidelines for the content and time frame of the report. Such agencies include departments of elder affairs, social services, health and welfare, human resources, or public health. Many of these agencies provide 24-hour hotline coverage, which enables immediate reporting.

In some states, mandatory reporting laws clearly state who is to be contacted in the event that elder abuse is suspected. There may be reporting hotlines or offices that

assume the responsibility for accepting the referral. Thobaben and Anderson (1985) have summarized national reporting laws and provide a chart that lists when reporting
must occur as well as when investigations must be conducted. This chart is reproduced in Table 7-1. It is important to note that mandatory reporters need not *prove* that
abuse or neglect has occurred; however, they are expected
to call in cases they feel are *suspicious* for abuse or neglect.
The verification of such cases is up to the state agency
responsible for accepting the referred suspected elder abuse
cases.

Verification is probably the most difficult and judgmental
step in the process of determining elder abuse and often
takes the most time. It is also an area that may seemingly
overlap with issues of malpractice, as in cases when elderly
nursing home residents are found to be severely dehydrated
or overmedicated.

After a referred elder has gone through the initial screening process, the health care practitioner will need to explore
the nature and circumstances of the precipitating event, in
order to provide the necessary information to appropriate
officials or administrative personnel. This can prove difficult as well, as there is a wide range in what is required from
one jurisdiction to another.

Salend, Kane, Satz, and Pynoos (1984, p. 61) conclude
that, "generally, the statutes have failed to ensure consistent information about elder abuse within or across states."
The content of the statutes they analyzed was found to vary
widely in purpose, coverage, implementation, agency, regis-
try requirements, mandated reporters, and reporting requirements. Provisions for immunity, confidentiality, investigation, and service also varied.

Table 7-2, reprinted from Salend et al. (1984), summarizes the typical state experiences in developing and implementing elder abuse statutes and highlights important areas
for consideration, with specific examples of state experiences. Of particular interest are the referral sources, types

of cases, substantiation rates, court-related activities, and prosecution activity. The referral sources indicate that, while there were reports received from both community members and professionals, there were more reports received from the community than originally expected. The Massachusetts state reporting agencies bear these findings out. It has been documented by the Massachusetts Executive Office of Elder Affairs (EOEA) that professionals account for only a small percentage of reports. People in the community are most likely to report suspected cases of elder abuse or neglect. This may be because professionals are likely to explore the nature of the event more thoroughly before making a report, often deciding that the situation does not warrant a report. Another possibility is they may put a care plan in place which remedies the situation and makes them feel they have met their obligation to the victim. Decision making in reporting elder abuse will be discussed in more detail later in the chapter.

The types of cases noted in Table 7-2 are another interesting finding from this study. Cases of neglect are the highest percentage of cases reported, followed by physical abuse and financial exploitation. Again, the Massachusetts EOEA reports similar findings (Glickman, Jakubiak, & Boynton, 1985). In fiscal year 1985, out of a total of 1,816 abuse reports made to the EOEA, fully 742 (41%) were classified as neglect cases, while 454 (25%) were classified as emotional abuse and 620 (34%) were labeled physical abuse. The EOEA also reports that the "neglect" case victim is most likely to be in the worst physical condition and most likely to die as a result of the neglect. The table denotes that cases of self-neglect comprise the majority of neglect cases; however, this is not borne out by the EOEA figures from Massachusetts, where "self-neglect" is not covered under the statutes.

Substantiation rates (substantiation means alleged cases that are *proven*) are noted to be "often unavailable" or "kept only at the county level," with a range of from 20 to 80

TABLE 7-1 Reporting Elder Abuse: A Summary from the States

State	Coverage for Whom	Physical Mistreatment	Mental Anguish	Neglect	Exploitation
Alabama (1)	18+•	X	X	X	X
Alaska (2)	65+	X	X	X	Financial
Arizona (3)	•	X		X	X
Arkansas (4)	18+•	X	X	X	X
California (5)	65+	X	X	X	X
Colorado (6)	65+•	X		X	X
Connecticut (7)	60+	X	X	X	X
Delaware (8)	18+•				X
Florida (9)	•	X	X	X	X
Georgia (10)	18+•	X	X	X	X

Other Abuses Covered	Reporting When[a]	Penalty for Failure[b]	Investigation When
	Immediate verbal, then written	B, C, D	Required within 3 days of report
	Within 24 hrs	B	To begin promptly; including personal interview
	Immediate verbal; written in 48 hrs	B	As soon as possible
	Immediate verbal; written in 48 hrs	B, E	Not defined
Abandonment	Immediate verbal; written in 36 hrs	B, C	Not defined*
Confinement, intimidation	Immediate written	—	Immediately if adult consents in writing
Abandonment	Within 5 days	B, C	Prompt evaluation, including home visit by ombudsman*
	—	—	Prompt and thorough
	Immediate verbal; written in 48 hrs	B	Immediate*
	—	B	Prompt and thorough, including a home visit*

(Continued)

TABLE 7–1 (Continued)

State	Coverage for Whom	Physical Mistreatment	Mental Anguish	Neglect	Exploitation
Hawaii (11)	65+	Actual or threatened	X	X	
Idaho (12)	60+	X	X	X	X
Illinois (13)	60+	X			Financial
Iowa (15)	18+•	X		X	X
Kentucky (17)	18+•	X	X	X	X
Louisiana (18)	18+	X	X	X	X
Maine (19)	18+•	X	X	X	X
Massachusetts (21)†	60+	X			
Michigan (22)	18+	X	X	X	X
Minnesota (23)	18+•	X	X	X	

†In Massachusetts each form of abuse is covered and investigation must occur within 24 hours or, if urgent, immediately.

Other Abuses Covered	Reporting When[a]	Penalty for Failure[b]	Investigation When
	Immediate verbal, then written	—	Action toward preventing further abuse within 24 hrs, when appropriate*
Abandonment	Within 24 hrs		Prompt and thorough evaluation of report*
	—	—	—
	—	—	Adult to be examined in 1 hr for immediate physical threat; otherwise, within 24 hrs
	Immediate verbal or written	B, C	As soon as possible*
Extortion	Immediate verbal, then written	B, C, D	Prompt, including interview and home visit if possible
Confinement	Immediate verbal; written in 48 hrs	Licensing board notified; C	—
	Immediately	B, C	—
	Immediate verbal	E	Within 24 hrs
	Immediate verbal, then written	B, E	Immediate

(Continued)

TABLE 7–1 (Continued)

State	Coverage for Whom	Physical Mistreatment	Mental Anguish	Neglect	Exploitation
Missouri (25)	60+•	Risk			
Montana (26)	60+	X	X	X	X
Nebraska (27)	•	X		X	
Nevada (28)	60+	X		X	X
New Hampshire (29)	18+•	X	X	X	X
New Mexico (31)	55+	X		X	X
N. Carolina (33)	18+•	X	X	X	X
Ohio (35)	60+•	X	X	X	X
Oklahoma (36)	65+	X		X	Financial
Oregon (37)	65+	X		X	
Rhode Island (39)	60+	X		X	X
S. Carolina (40)	18+•	X		X	X
Tennessee (42)	18+•	X	X	X	X

Other Abuses Covered	Reporting When[a]	Penalty for Failure[b]	Investigation When
	—	—	Prompt and thorough
	—	B	—
	Verbal, then written	B	Immediate, if warranted by report
	Immediate verbal	B	Within 3 days
Confinement	Immediate verbal, then written	B	Within 3 days*
	Promptly	B	Immediate*
	—	—	Prompt and thorough including home visit*
	Immediate verbal or written	—	Within 24 hrs in an emergency; otherwise within 3 working days*
	Prompt oral	B	Prompt and thorough*
Abandonment	Immediate verbal	B, C	Prompt
Abandonment	Immediately	B, C	Immediate
Confinement	Immediate verbal	B, C, D	Within 3 days
	Immediately	B, C, D	As soon as possible; reporter notified of determination*

(*Continued*)

TABLE 7–1 (Continued)

State	Coverage for Whom	Physical Mistreatment	Mental Anguish	Neglect	Exploitation
Texas (43)	65+•	X	X	X	X
Utah (44)	18+•	X		X	X
Vermont (45)	60+	X		X	X
Virginia (46)	18+•	X	X	X	X
Washington (47)	60+•	X	X	X	X
West Virginia (48)	18+•	X		X	
Wisconsin (49)	60+•	X		X	Material
Wyoming (50)	•	X		X	X

Key: •   Physically or mentally impaired
     ——   Not specified
      *   Consent required for services to allegedly abused elder
[a]Reporting is voluntary, not mandatory, in four states: Colorado, Iowa, Wisconsin, and Wyoming. Nine states have no "in home" adult abuse reporting law: Indiana (14), Kansas (16), Maryland (20), Mississippi (24), New Jersey (30), New York (32), North Dakota (34), Pennsylvania (38), and South Dakota (41).

Other Abuses Covered	Reporting When[a]	Penalty for Failure[b]	Investigation When
—	—	—	Within 24 hrs*
Confinement	Immediately	B —	—*
	Verbal, then written in 1 wk	B, C	Within 72 hrs
Abandonment	Immediately	—	Prompt, including home visit and consultation with relevant others
Abandonment	Immediate verbal, then written	—	—*
	Immediately	B, C, D	—
—	—	—	Within 24 hrs
—	—	—	—

[b]Codes for penalties:
 A = Report filed with department named in reference
 B = Misdemeanor
 C = Fine, ranging from $25 to $1,000
 D = Imprisonment, ranging from 10 days to 6 months
 E = Civil liability for damages due to failure to report

Source: M. Thobaben & L. Anderson. Reporting Elder Abuse: It's the Law. *American Journal of Nursing*, 85(4), 1985, 371–374. Reprinted with permission of Marshelle Thobaben, R.N., M.S., and Linda Anderson, R.N., M.N., both associate professors in the Department of Nursing of Humboldt State University, Arcata, CA, and the *American Journal of Nursing*.

TABLE 7–2 Typical State Experiences in Developing and Implementing Elder Abuse Reporting Statutes

Areas of Consideration	Prototype State Experiences
Impetus for progress of the laws	Need perceived by direct service providers (social workers, nurses, home health aides) No formal needs assessment; anecdotal evidence Legislative support sought by professional coalitions Child abuse reporting laws and adult abuse reporting laws of other states used as models
Purpose of laws	To provide statutory authority to social service departments and define their responsibility To protect those in need through mechanism for state intervention To provide guidelines for workers in case investigation and service delivery
Structure of reporting systems	Reports usually received at county level Reports investigated promptly Reports usually received in state and local departments of social services, adult services units
Referral sources	Reports received from both community and professionals More reports received from community than originally expected
Number of cases reported	Number of reports has increased each year since passage of laws Number of reports has been greater than expected Statistical breakdown of elderly cases often unavailable
Types of cases	Cases of neglect were highest percentage of cases reported; next largest category was physical abuse, followed by financial exploitation

TABLE 7–2 (Continued)

Areas of Consideration	Prototype State Experiences
	Cases of self-neglect comprised majority of neglect cases
	Typical abuse case thought to involve caretaker suffering from financial and emotional stress
Substantiation rates	Often unavailable or kept only at county level
	Range of 20-80% substantiation rate
Court-related activity	Few court petitions, usually 1-2% of total caseload; few services provided involuntarily
Court-related activity	Cases must be very serious for court intervention; legal remedies are last resort; majority of court petitions are granted
Prosecution activity	Little or no prosecution of alleged abusers or those failing to report
	Few successful prosecutions
Funding for adult protective services	Perceived inadequacy of funding
	Bias toward child welfare services
	Adult protective services allocated low percentage of total Title XX funds
	Many states severely underfunded

Source: E. Salend, R. Kane, M. Satz, & J. Pynoos. Elder Abuse Reporting: Limitations of Statutes. *The Gerontologist,* 24(1), 1984, 61-69, Table 1. Reprinted by permission of *The Gerontologist.*

percent (Salend et al., 1984). In Massachusetts, the substantiation rate averages around 70 percent for the EOEA, which is responsible for community-dwelling elders, while it averages around 45 percent for the Department of Public Health (DPH), which is responsible for nursing home cases. In any event, the variation in substantiation rates is an issue that warrants further examination. To date, there are no studies that account for the varying rates of substantiation among reported cases.

Finally, the court-related and prosecution activities listed in Table 7-2 are extremely provocative. Salend et al. (1984) report that alleged abusers or those failing to report are rarely if ever prosecuted and that such lawsuits are seldom successful. There are few court petitions, and cases must be "serious" for court intervention. These findings appear to be consistent with reporting and prosecution for other forms of family violence. It is interesting to note that, for all the emotion abuse-reporting laws evoke, there are really very few "teeth" in such laws. Clearly, much more research is needed in the area of reporting, in order to improve the legal system and its benefits to elders. Because there is no federal legislation, the individuality of state reporting laws will continue to pose difficulty for those studying reporting patterns and outcomes across states.

METHODS OF COLLECTING DATA FOR REPORTS

What mechanisms are being utilized for the collection of the elder abuse and neglect data so often cited in the literature? Most states use some type of standardized intake form, in combination with an assessment form that guides protective service workers in their investigations. Table 7-3 provides as an example the intake form utilized by the Massachusetts EOEA. The actual investigation form is much longer and can be found in its entirety in Appendix B. An argument can be made that the investigation form is excessive and unnecessarily burdensome for the protective service worker who is charged with its implementation. However, a case can also be made for obtaining as much data as possible in order to consider as many factors in the alleged event as possible. Until more is known about the phenomenon of elder abuse and neglect, it is likely that health care professionals who call in such cases will have to collect a large amount of information in order to report a case.

TABLE 7–3 Elder Abuse Mandated Reporter Form, Massachusetts EOEA

This form should be returned within 48 hours of the oral report.

Reporter Information:
  Name: _____
  Occupation: _____
  Agency: _____
  Address: _____
  Tel. #: _____

Information about Alleged Victim:
  Name: _____
  Address: _____
  Permanent: _____
  Temporary: _____
  Tel. #: _____
  Approximate Age: _____ Sex: _____ Language: _____

Information about Alleged Abuser:
  Name: _____
  Address: _____
  Tel. # _____
  Relationship to Elder: _____

Type of Abuse Reported (include nature and extent):
  Physical: _____ Emotional: _____ Neglect: _____
  Describe: _____
  _____
  _____
  _____

Is reporter aware of prior injuries, abuse or neglect? Yes ____ No ____

If yes, indicate nature of incident and date if known: _____
_____
_____
_____

Is medical treatment required immediately? Yes ___ No ___ Possibly ___
Describe treatment needed or already received: _____
_____
_____
_____

Does reporter believe the situation constitutes an emergency? Yes ___
No ___ Possibly ___

(Continued)

TABLE 7-3 (Continued)

Describe the risk of death or immediate and serious harm: _____

_____

_____

_____

How did reporter first become aware of the alleged injuries? _____

_____

_____

Information about caretaker, relatives, and other persons or agencies
knowledgeable of the alleged victim:
Name   Agency/Relationship Caretaker   Address   Tel. #

_____

_____

_____

Additional information or comments:

_____

_____

_____

_____

Signature of Reporter	Date

THE PROCESS OF DECIDING TO REPORT

Let us now discuss in more detail the decision-making process that leads an individual to report a suspected case of
elder abuse or neglect.

Phillips and Rempusheski (1985, 1986) have conducted
studies examining the phenomenon of decision making in
elder abuse reporting, utilizing grounded theory technique
to formulate a four-stage decision-making model. Tape-
recorded interviews of a sample of 29 health care providers
(16 nurses and 13 social workers) were coded and analyzed.
The research questions that were central to these studies
were:

1. How do health care providers giving advice and care to the elderly in the community conceptualize elder abuse and neglect?
2. How do health care providers translate their definitions of elder abuse and neglect into decisions about abused and/or neglected elders?
3. What social phenomena surround health care providers' decision-making processes for elder abuse and neglect?
4. What other characteristics of elders and caregivers enhance or inhibit health care providers' decisions regarding the presence or absence of elder abuse and neglect?

The authors state that "the model shows that health care providers assess the quality of care-giving situations and not the quality of elder-caregiver relationships when making decisions about abuse and neglect" (Phillips & Rempusheski, 1985, p. 135). Decisions about elder abuse or neglect are influenced by both the caregiver's overall knowledge of the elder's needs and the caregiver's ability to meet those needs. If a caregiver is frail and debilitated, as in the case of a 75-year-old daughter caring for a 95-year-old mother, the health care professional is most likely to label it a "bad situation" but not abuse or neglect. The same holds true when a care provider is incapacitated by a personal or health problem such as mental retardation, alcoholism, drug addiction, or psychiatric disease. It seems that health care providers are also influenced by the perceived amount of effort that is being spent on a given situation. When a caregiver seems to be trying hard to provide good care to an elder, an abuse or neglect label is unlikely, even if actions or inactions result in serious injury to the elder. Finally, the elder's personality enters into the decision-making process. If an elder is perceived by a health care professional as exceedingly demanding or difficult to get along with, the situation is less likely to be perceived as abuse or neglect. The findings from this study seem to indicate that there is a variety of value-decisions that are being made in deciding whether or not an event should be labeled abuse or neglect. The health care professional brings to the situation a set of personal values, cultural stereotypes, and professional values that influence the perception of the event.

While this study focuses on community-dwelling elders only, it has been our experience that the same issues are relevant to the institutional setting. When a long-term-care facility expresses concern and affection for an elder who is being evaluated for suspected elder abuse or neglect, the acute-care health professional is less likely to perceive a set of signs and symptoms as elder abuse or neglect. The following is a case in point.

> Mrs. R was admitted to the intensive care unit via the emergency unit for a pneumothorax that was the result of a fractured rib sustained during a fall. She also had numerous hematomas on her upper arms and torso. She had a long history of dementia and was known to wander. The health professionals in the acute-care facility were initially very concerned that the woman had been neglected. How else could such an event happen? The long-term-care facility "must have known" she was a high risk for such an injury, and they were responsible for her safety. Perhaps they had been lax in their supervision.
>
> The nurse from the intensive-care unit called the facility and was immediately impressed by the caring and concern voiced by the nurse she spoke to. Mrs. R had lived at the facility for 19 years and was a "favorite" among the staff. Apparently, during change of shift, she had managed to unlock her wheelchair and roll it through an exit to the stairs. She had fallen to the next landing, where she was discovered. The severity of her injuries were consistent with the story, and the acute-care-facility nurse now saw the event as an "accident" instead of neglect.

This case illustrates how personal values and perceptions influence decision making in determining whether a situation should be labeled abuse or neglect. The legal system might argue that, regardless of intention, the situation was clearly one of negligence. We know, however, that a large number of events very similar to this one will never reach the courts, primarily because the decision-making process as carried out by health care professionals often halts a report before it gets to state agencies and lawmakers.

Some health care professionals argue that the label *elder abuse* or *neglect* is a dangerous one in that it overlaps with poor professional care. "Bad doctoring," such as the prescription of multiple diuretics that, when poorly monitored, can ultimately lead to dehydration and serious fluid and electrolyte imbalance, is an example. If, prior to the passage of elder abuse reporting laws, an elderly person who suffers an injury due to inadequate care already was protected by malpractice suits, perhaps we are doing a disservice to the elderly by creating a new category called elder abuse. Callahan (1981) reminds us that public definitions are important and do change behavior: "When alcoholism was called a crime, people went to jail. When it was called a disease, people went to drying out facilities" (p. 3). If, by creating a new category, we deflect a case that should have been prosecuted as malpractice, we have done a grave disservice to our elderly. Those in the legal profession will need to pay attention to trends that evolve as a result of mandatory elder abuse and neglect reporting laws.

FOLLOW-UP ON REPORTED CASES

Once a case of suspected elder abuse or neglect has been reported, what follow-up mechanisms are in place to insure the situation does not recur? Here lies a problem in the system. As Cohen (1984) describes it, in most states, the process of follow-up that occurs immediately after a report involves an investigation that must be initiated within a 24-hour period and must reach a conclusion either verifying or disclaiming a report in a timely manner. Most states also require that a service plan be initiated immediately if a referred case is corroborated.

These short-term measures are not enough, however, and less is known about follow-up in the long run. How long is the state responsible for following the elder abuse or neglect victim's case? How long should special services be provided by one state agency when there are other state and federal programs that provide similar services? What is the role of family members who could provide services to elders? What is the role of the acute-care facility regarding long-term follow-up? These are difficult questions that are as yet unanswered. If there is no process for monitoring a situation, the abuse or neglect event may occur again. Health care professionals should incorporate a follow-up plan of care when they suspect and report a case of elder abuse. This may be accompanied by telephone contact, VNA referral, home visit, or calling a next-door neighbor who is familiar with the situation. A successful follow-up program is essential for the prevention of future abuse or neglect.

REFERENCES

Callahan, J. J. (1981, March 23–25, April 1–3). *Elder Abuse Programming— Will It Help the Elderly?* Paper presented at the National Conference on the Abuse of Older Persons. Boston and San Francisco.

Cohen, E. S. (1984, September). Elder Abuse. *The Coordinator*, 12–60.

Glickman, L., Jakubiak, C., & Boynton, K. (1985). *Program Report: Elder Protective Services, July 1, 1983–June 30, 1985.* Boston: Executive Office of Elder Affairs, Commonwealth of Massachusetts.

Oakar, M. R., & Miller, C. A. (1983). Federal Legislation to Protect the Elderly. In J. I. Kosberg (Ed.), *Abuse and Maltreatment of the Elderly: Causes and Interventions.* Littleton, MA: PSG Publishing.

Phillips, L. R., & Rempusheski, V. F. (1985). A Decision-Making Model for Diagnosing and Intervening in Elder Abuse and Neglect. *Nursing Research, 34*(3), 134–139.

Phillips, L. R., & Rempusheski, V. F. (1986). Making Decisions about Elder Abuse. *Social Casework, 67*(3), 131–140.

Salend, E., Kane, R., Satz, M., & Pynoos, J. (1984). Elder Abuse Reporting: Limitations of Statutes. *The Gerontologist, 24*(1), 61–69.

Thobaben, M., & Anderson, L. (1985). Reporting Elder Abuse: It's the Law. *American Journal of Nursing, 85*(4), 371–374.

U.S. House of Representatives, Select Committee on Aging. (1979, June 23). *Elder Abuse: The Hidden Problem.* Washington, DC: U.S. Government Printing Office.

8

Ethical Issues

Ethical issues are rampant in cases of suspected elder abuse and neglect. They pose great difficulty for health care workers who are trying to intervene effectively and frequently. Ethical dilemmas identified in any given case are rather discipline specific, as illustrated in the following case quoted from Wetle (1986).

> Ms. B lived for many years with her brother, who had a history of multiple hospitalizations for schizophrenia. Because of her own frail health and problems with mobility, Ms. B had not been out of her apartment for more than five years, depending totally upon her brother for shopping and errands. When her brother was hospitalized once again because of his bizarre behavior, including an assault on a neighbor, the landlord began eviction proceedings and called a local agency to seek assistance with Ms. B. The landlord's concern for Ms. B's welfare was, in part, due to the stench of garbage coming from the apartment. In addition, he reported that no one had been in or out of her apartment in more than a week. A social worker was dispatched to evaluate the situation but was initially refused entry to Ms. B's apartment. Eventually, on the third try, Ms. B agreed to talk with the social worker but refused to accept any needed services except for a legal aid attorney to fight the eviction. A week later, Ms. B fell and was hospitalized. The attending physician, alarmed at her physical condition, had Ms. B sent to a

nursing home to protect her from further harm. The social worker was angry with the attorney for not fighting institutionalization of Ms. B and angry with the physician for not considering community-based alternatives. The physician was angry with the social worker for blatantly neglecting Ms. B's needs. The attorney was angry with the physician for not consulting her regarding the placement.

Each of the professionals involved in this case had a different perspective and approach to Ms. B. The social worker, trained to act as an advocate in seeking assistance for the client, even when the client refused assistance, hoped that by early intervention a more serious and perhaps irreversible crisis might be avoided. The attorney's role was to execute the client's wishes as the client expressed them. The physician, believing that the patient's competence was compromised, wanted to protect the patient from further harm. Each was acting within the ethical code of his or her own profession; each was trying to do what was "right" for the patient. [pp. 261–262][1]

While the "right" action is not always clear, it is fair to say that the majority of health care professionals are sincerely concerned about the health and well-being of their elderly patients. When confronted with a case of blatant abuse or neglect, they often react with outrage and express a desire to obtain some kind of justice for the elder. There is also usually a desire to protect the elderly person from further mistreatment, which may take the form of paternalistic decision making for the elder and/or the enforcement of an unsolicited protective service system plan. Paternalism often arises out of good intentions. Health care providers intend to protect the elderly they care for, but, in doing so, they may make decisions *for* instead of *with* the older person. This frequently results in actions that would not be consistent with the usual choice the elder would make.

---

[1]*Source*: T. T. Wetle, Ethical Aspects of Decision Making for and with the Elderly. In M. B. Kapp, H. E. Pies, & A. E. Doudera (Eds.), *Legal and Ethical Aspects of Health Care for the Elderly* (pp. 258–267). Ann Arbor, MI: University of Michigan, Health Administration Press, 1986. Reprinted with permission.

Protective service system plans also usually arise out of good intentions, but there has been much public criticism in our country regarding such services for adults. This is usually based on whether or not the state has legal authority to intervene unilaterally in the private life of an unwilling elder. Kapp (1986) states that "health care professionals have an essential role to play in appropriate circumstances in encouraging their competent older patients (and almost all patients are competent for most of their lives) to accept, voluntarily, intelligently, and thoughtfully, necessary and available protective services, on either a present or future basis" (p. 233). This is not meant to imply that paternalism should be employed in order to convince elders that it is in their best interest to accept whatever plan is offered. Paternalism can be detrimental in that it can be insulting, ineffective, and even harmful when an individual's rights are not respected. Most health care professionals, however, have been rightfully accused of paternalistic behavior when they have honestly been trying to be helpful. Wetle (1986) states that, "ideally, there should be no ethical issues unique to decision making and the elderly. Once one has left childhood, age in and of itself should have no influence on the ethics involved in decision making regarding treatment, nontreatment, and the distribution of health-care resources" (p. 258).

At each step in the process of managing elderly persons who manifest signs of inadequate care, there are ethical issues. Table 8–1 indicates the most significant ethical issues at each stage of the process of case management. The following discussion will deal with each of these.

ISSUES IN IDENTIFYING AND REPORTING CASES

There are significant differences in the appropriateness and usefulness of definitions that are to be used to estimate the incidence or prevalence of abuse and neglect in the general population versus those definitions that are required to

TABLE 8-1 Ethical Issues in Various Stages of Case Management

Stage	Ethical Issues
Identifying and reporting cases	Purpose of identification Effects of labeling *Primum non nocere* Confidentiality
Gaining access	Strategies Right to privacy Responsibility if access refused
Intervening	Paternalism Self-determination vs. dependency Right to be abused Incompetency of the elderly person
Ongoing responsibility	Contact vs. abandonment Minimized risk Free and informed consent

identify cases for further intervention or legal sanctions. Ethical dilemmas can result when there is discrepancy between the definitional elements of abuse or neglect and the perceived needs of the elder. The difficulty arises because the broader definitions that have been used to estimate the prevalence of the problem have been used as well to trigger a response from the protective service system. Unfortunately, these definitions are not precise enough to discriminate between cases of abuse and neglect that warrant legal/ criminal proceedings and cases of neglect that result in inadequate care and in which there is no intentional injury.

The issues the elder abuse reporter must sort out are the nature, extent, and intentionality of the situation, as well as the reasonableness of the situation in light of the resources and level of accountability the care provider can be held to. In cases of intentional physical abuse that result in trauma to the elder, few professionals would argue the validity of the label "elder abuse." However, when an elderly individual

presents who has been cared for at home by well-inten-
tioned family members who are inept because they are not
educated to be responsible for such symptoms as urine
burns and decubitus ulcers, the determination of abuse is
not clear.

Because the consequences are significant if one errone-
ously identifies a case as abuse and neglect when it is not,
the definitions used to identify cases for intervention must
be different from those used in population studies. They
must be very precise and designed to include only the most
flagrant cases. Unfortunately, this is seldom the case with
the current abuse statutes. *Primum non nocere* (above all do no
harm) is an essential guide in these situations. The health
care professional must be aware of the potential harm that
could result from inappropriately labeling someone as a
victim of abuse and neglect. Possible detrimental effects
include

- Social stigma with resultant loss of support from
  friends and community
- Loss of autonomy
- Disruption of home life
- Loss of nursing home bed
- Expense of potential legal proceedings
- Inappropriate criminal sanctions

The use of inappropriate definitions results in two problems that in turn can pose ethical dilemmas for the practitioner. The first is that, by too narrowly defining abuse and
neglect and limiting intervention to only those cases, we
exclude from care a large number of elderly persons who
experience inadequate care (which is not abuse) who could
benefit from intervention. If they are competing for limited
resources, these elderly might not receive services. The
second problem occurs when a broad definition forces the
inclusion of cases that cannot be appropriately managed
using the interventions mandated by law. In such an instance, it is possible that the act of reporting such a case,

although mandated, could cause potential harm to the elderly person or family.

The following case illustrates the dilemma that arises when inadequate care requiring a social/medical intervention is identified. Reporting it would trigger a criminal/legal system response designed to address a broad definition of abuse and neglect. The issue is whether or not this case should be reported for possible criminal sanctions because of neglect resulting in serious injury.

A 78-year-old woman who had suffered a severe stroke and had resultant dense left hemiparesis was cared for at home by her husband of 50 years who was limited by severe osteoarthritis of the hips. He was able to assist her adequately with bathing, grooming, dressing, and feeding until she sustained a partial right hemiparesis and became totally bedridden. Her husband continued to try to provide all of her care, but over several weeks she developed multiple decubitus ulcers, became malnourished, and was ultimately brought to the emergency room when she was unresponsive because of severe dehydration and pyelonephritis.

According to the definitions given in the first chapter of this book, this is a case of neglect in which serious harm resulted because of the failure to provide adequate care. There is a victim; however, there is no crime in the sense of intentional injury. The real question is whether reporting this case will help resolve the inadequate care. It is unlikely that any statute that defines this case as a crime could be applied beneficially. Indeed, it is likely that the husband would be labeled as a "wife neglecter." It is possible that he could be fined or even imprisoned, but it is unlikely that the criminal justice system would be prepared to direct the types of services that could resolve the wife's inadequate care. The ethical issue of whether to report a case such as this must rest with the caretaker's assessment of the risks and benefits that such a report may have on the elderly person. Inappropriately labeling a case of inadequate care as abuse and neglect may be hazardous to a patient's health.

The allegation of "abuse" is a powerful one. Once an elder abuse referral has been made, the elder is often referred to as "the abuse case" long before any investigatory work has been done. Labeling a person "abused" is a serious charge, and it may be wiser to use a totally different nomenclature in order to prevent such a label. Family members, visitors, and other patients may overhear the word "abuse" and have strong reactions to it. Discretion is very important when dealing with such a sensitive issue.

Another issue in identification and reporting concerns confidentiality of the information exchanged between the health professional and the patient. The American Medical Association (AMA) code holds that "a physician may not reveal the confidences entrusted to him in the course of medical attendance, or the deficiencies he may observe in the character of his patients, unless he is required to do so by law, or unless it becomes necessary in order to protect the welfare of the individual or of the community" (AMA, 1951; see also Beauchamp & Childress, 1983, p. 25). Nursing and social work professionals follow similar codes within their professions. When there is a conflict between legally mandated reporting requirements and the confidentiality of doctor-patient communications, it is important to keep the patient's welfare uppermost. If the potential harm of reporting is significant and the indications for reporting are marginal, then the practitioner should probably not report the case. This is usually possible without fear of legal reprisals because most reporting laws leave discretion to the practitioner as to whether there is "reason to believe" that abuse or neglect has occurred.

In situations where the potential harm to the elderly person from inadequate care outweighs the potential harm from reporting the case, the health care professional should explain the rationale to the elder and make every effort to get his or her approval to make a report. In actual practice, it is often possible to discuss the issue of reporting with the elder in a way that gains his or her acquiescence. It is particularly useful to emphasize that the elder will retain control of the timing and extent of any interventions and that no substantive changes can or will be made without the elder's acceptance.

ISSUES IN GAINING ACCESS

The issue of access raises several difficult ethical issues involving strategies for gaining access, the elderly person's right to privacy, and the proper response to being refused entry. In order to gain access to the elderly person effectively, one must use a strategy that permits voluntary involvement by the elder and offers positive benefit to that person, such as improved shelter or nutritional supplements on a regular basis. It is at this critical juncture that the impact of inappropriate definitions is felt the most.

Very few elderly persons want or are willing to accept help for "abuse and neglect." The terms imply wrongdoing on the part of a family member or some inherent defect in the elderly person that makes them "deserve" abuse and neglect. The effects of labeling must be remembered at all times. If health professionals choose to use these terms, then it is unlikely that they will successfully negotiate access. Without voluntary access, no intervention is likely to be effective. It is imperative, then, that the health care professional avoid the term *abuse* and *neglect* when trying to negotiate access and rely instead on less negative terms such as *help with activities of daily living, closer attention to health needs, easier ways to get meals and medications and to go shopping,* and so forth. It is important to frame the problem in a manner that promotes the elderly person's willingness to recognize it and deal with it. To do otherwise is to cause inappropriate loss of the opportunity to intervene, which constitutes a professional failure to fulfill intended obligations to the patient.

Despite the professional's obligation to develop the most effective strategies, the elderly person has an unassailable right to privacy. Among other things, this means that there will never be unchallenged statutes that permit legislatively mandated access to elders against their will in their own homes. Other strategies that are based on negotiation are essential and more attractive, despite the professional's understandable desire to solve the difficult issue of access. The following is a case in point.

> A 67-year-old woman who lived alone was seen several times in the emergency room for contusions sustained in "falls." During one visit she stated that her injuries resulted from beatings by her drug-abusing grandson. During the previous three years she had been harrassed, threatened with injury, and beaten when she refused to give him money. She was not harmed when she acquiesced, but, whenever she tried to force him to stop, she was beaten. None of the other family members were able to modify his behavior, although neither the police nor the courts were involved. She adamantly refused to permit any outside help for what she termed "a family problem" and forbade the physician from reporting it. When it was reported, she refused access to the protective service workers. She continues to receive her medical care from her physician but refuses to discuss the status of her "family problem."

This case demonstrates one of the most frustrating situations that a health care worker can face: the responsibility of respecting every person's right to privacy, even where abuse is known to be occurring. At the same time, this does not necessarily mean that the professional must sit back and do nothing; in fact, there are continuing responsibilities that must be addressed when access is refused. These include developing alternative strategies for gaining access to the elder and developing strategies to influence the behavior of the caretaker/abuser.

Alternate strategies for gaining access include the use of nonthreatening medical personnel, such as visiting nurses, and the use of individuals known to the elder or their family. These individuals might include clergy, neighbors, relatives, and friends. Any one of these individuals might be able to provide an entree for the health care professional to initiate assessment and to begin the process of developing a relationship with the elder.

Similarly, these same individuals can also be used to attempt to influence the behavior of the caretaker/abuser. These attempts might include the threat of sanctions, an appeal to the individual's responsibilities for providing adequate care, or a suggestion that the caretaker/abuser seek supportive services himself. Occasionally it is possible to gain some degree of cooperation from the caretaker/abuser by threatening to put into jeopardy the income that comes to the caretaker/abuser through the elderly person. For example, by threatening to have Social Security or pension benefits held up because of the question of inadequate care, the health care professional can frequently gain access to the elder. This is often effective even though no such mechanism exists.

In summary, it is important for the health care professional to continue to seek innovative ways of gaining access to the elder either in the home or in the more controlled medical setting. Frequently this requires the participation of a large number of people.

ISSUES IN INTERVENING

Self-determination versus dependency is a central issue in intervention. There are often conflicting values between the practitioner and the elderly person, such as when the health care practitioner feels that the elderly person is in an unsafe situation and at risk for abuse or neglect but the elder does not wish to leave. It is often difficult for practitioners to see that they are imposing their concepts of what is an adequate goal of intervention on the elderly person. Despite the most laudable motives and the sincerest desire to eliminate the abuse or neglect, the health care professional cannot usurp the elder's right to decide what is in his or her best interest, even if the practitioner feels this is wrong. Consequently, it is appropriate to negotiate intervention with the elderly person, rather than try to make a professional prescription. The following case illustrates the process of negotiation.

Mrs. P was an alert and oriented 86-year-old woman who was admitted through the emergency unit for pneumonia and evaluation of bruises around her head, neck, and upper chest. She was ambulatory with assistance and needed help with her activities of daily living. She was living with her two adult sons at the time of admission, both of whom had known psychiatric histories. Mrs. P admitted that her bruises were inflicted by her sons, who became extremely agitated whenever she had an episode of incontinence. Outraged, the physician requested an elder abuse consultation and assured Mrs. P that he would see to it that an alternative living situation was arranged. Mrs. P was quick to refuse this alternative, stating that her sons were "good boys" and she would be going home with them.

After a great deal of negotiation between Mrs. P and the physician, it was agreed that an appropriate intermediate step would be to place a home health aide with her. While Mrs. P was not pleased with the idea initially, she did understand that it might decrease the chance of another episode of violence. Since her sons were especially unable to cope with her incontinence, it was explained that a home health aide would be able to help her with her toileting and hygiene. She was discharged to home with the assignment of a home health aide, and this arrangement has worked well. To Mrs. P, the issue was how to remain at home with her sons in a way that was most comfortable for all of them. Eliminating the abuse was not her primary goal. To her, the beatings were a reasonable price to pay for the benefits that she derived from being home with her sons. To the physician, the elimination of the abuse was the paramount issue.

In such a situation, it is important to remember that it is the elderly person who determines what can and should be done. It is helpful for the health care professional to ask whether the proposed interventions are more likely to respond to the professional's sense of outrage and paternalistic need to do something or to meeting the needs and desires of the elderly person. It is often difficult to acknowledge that any competent adult has the right "to be abused." This is an extreme position, but it reflects the individual's autonomy concerning his or her own care and welfare. Paternalism has been called "the most insidious loss of liberty for an elderly person" (Ratzan, 1983, p. 524), although it is understandably difficult to avoid in cases of inadequate care. The following case illustrates this problem.

Mrs. T was a frail widowed woman who had lived independently but with increasing difficulty, caring for herself, prior to an admission for atrial fibrillation, congestive heart failure, and a new dense left hemiparesis from an embolic stroke. Her daughter insisted that she be discharged to the daughter's home, despite Mrs. T's significant needs for assistance with personal care, toileting, and dressing. During the next several weeks Mrs. T's apartment was vacated and her belongings moved to her daughter's.

Over the following months a pattern of inadequate care emerged. Mrs. T missed or rescheduled most of her follow-up medical appointments. When examined she showed evidence of poor nutrition, contusions, and poorly controlled congestive heart failure. Despite a prescription for the same doses of digoxin and coumadin that had controlled her atrial fibrillation and provided adequate anticoagulation in the hospital, there were wide fluctuations in her heart rate and prothrombin times. Furthermore, her daughter began to refuse entry into the house to the home health aide and visiting nurse.

Mrs. T finally confided to the nurse that her daughter had started to drink heavily again and when drinking was physically and verbally abusive. In addition, she was very erratic in managing Mrs. T's complicated medication schedule. It became apparent that the major source of income for the family was Mrs. T's Social Security check, and her daughter refused to spend any of it for Mrs. T's medical needs. Initial attempts to confront the daughter with the consequences of her behavior only resulted in more resistance. Then Mrs. T's home health services were cut back due to a change in her insurance status, and her daughter refused to pay to restore the services to their previous level. This led to a hospitalization for congestive heart failure.

During this hospitalization, interventions were directed toward assisting the daughter with her own feelings of guilt, stress, and unmet needs. At the insistence of both mother and daughter, Mrs. T was again discharged home to the care of her daughter, despite the opinion of the medical team that she could be better cared for in a long-term-care facility. She receives home health services, and her daughter receives counseling support. Her inadequate care has not been eliminated, but it is less frequent.

This case was particularly distressing to the professionals involved because it was not always clear that Mrs. T was making uncoerced decisions. Although everyone felt that her inadequate care could not be eliminated unless she were institutionalized, they also realized that nursing home placement caused her more fear than remaining at home with her undependable daughter. Because the patient and daughter refused to consider any options other than care at home, the health care team responded by doing as much as possible within the limits of intervention set by the patient. Although the inadequate care was not eliminated and episodes of abuse and neglect continue, the patient prefers this to being in a nursing home. It is important for the health care professional to participate in any way that ultimately benefits the elderly. In this case, marginally inadequate care was the only alternative to dangerously inadequate care.

ONGOING RESPONSIBILITY

Most of the cases we have discussed in this chapter are examples of elderly persons or their families acting against the recommendations and wishes of health care professionals. Together they raise another important ethical obligation faced by health care workers. Despite the fact that there is a "right to be abused," and even when the elderly person exercises that right, health care professionals are not thereby relieved from their obligation to assure optimum care for that person. It is not appropriate for health care professionals to abandon the elderly person who rejects their plan of care. Attempts must be made to maintain contact with the individual, however tenuous. This is not only to monitor the progress, or lack of progress, but also to permit the continued negotiation of a care plan with the elderly person, in order to lessen the risk of further harm. It also affords the opportunity to provide those services that are acceptable to the family and the elderly person (such as a home health aide, meals on wheels, a visiting nurse, and so forth). There is an ethical obligation to see that some outside involvement is maintained with the elderly person.

There is the further obligation to assure that those elderly persons who do exercise their "right to be abused" do so without coercion by the person responsible for the abuse and with the full knowledge of the consequences and the available alternatives. Anything less than this could be considered inadequate care on the part of the professional.

REFERENCES

Beauchamp, T. L., & Childress, J. F. (1983). Confidentiality. In N. Abrams & M. Buckner (Eds.), *Medical Ethics* (pp. 23–27). Cambridge, MA: MIT Press.

Kapp, M. B. (1986). Adult Protective Services: Convincing the Patient to Consent. In M. B. Kapp, H. E. Pies, & A. E. Doudera (Eds.), *Legal and Ethical Aspects of Health Care for the Elderly* (pp. 231–244). Ann Arbor: University of Michigan, Health Administration Press.

Ratzan, R. M. (1983). Being Old Makes You Different: The Ethics of Research with Elderly Subjects. In N. Abrams & M. Buckner (Eds.), *Medical Ethics* (pp. 518–531). Cambridge, MA: MIT Press.

Wetle, T. T. (1986). Ethical Aspects of Decision Making for and with the Elderly. In M. B. Kapp, H. E. Pies, & A. E. Doudera (Eds.), *Legal and Ethical Aspects of Health Care for the Elderly* (pp. 258–267). Ann Arbor: University of Michigan, Health Administration Press.

9

Looking Ahead: Applying Theory to Practice

Clinicians and theoreticians alike share the common goals of preventing abuse, neglect, or inadequate care and of identifying them at the earliest stage possible. These goals are a focal point of activity to which both groups can contribute. The success of programs dedicated to prevention and early intervention in cases of inadequate care will lie in the clinician's ability to apply successfully what has been learned from research to the clinical setting. It is clear that theory in elder abuse and neglect has advanced to a stage where it now needs to be tested by health care practitioners. It seems appropriate that the majority of clinical activities should involve the identification of high risk elders in order to prevent inadequate care. The growing body of theoretical knowledge now provides justification for a number of interventions currently in use, and can provide guidance for further action.

Table 9-1 provides a framework for discussion that decribes the elder's place of residence as it relates to issues of theory and prevention. The purpose of this chapter is not to restate discussions of theory that have been presented in

We would like to express our appreciation to Karl Pillemer, Ph.D., of the University of New Hampshire for his helpful review of this chapter.

TABLE 9–1 Theoretical Models of Inadequate Care by Elder's Place of Residence

	Impairment theories (dependency of)	Stressed caretaker theory	Psychopathology of abuser theory	Transgenerational violence theory (cycle of violence)	Social isolation theory
Elders at home alone	—	—	—	—	—
Elders at home with others					
a) caregivers	X	X	X	X	X
b) noncaregivers	—	—	X	X	X
Institutional settings					
a) rest homes	X	X	X	X	—
b) nursing homes	X	X	X	X	—
c) hospitals	X	X	X	X	—

Chapter 2, but to use this grid for proposing interventions and solutions for inadequate care.

ELDERS AT HOME ALONE

Most studies of abuse and neglect include few elderly persons who live alone. It is unclear whether this is due to a lower incidence of abuse or (self) neglect in this group, differential reporting, or failure of these persons to meet the study definitions of abuse and neglect. These elderly persons are at risk for inadequate care through the failure to engage with existing service systems. The barriers that prevent this are often internal to the elderly person as well as due to the constraints of the service system and include ignorance of services, inability to access services, under reporting of illness and disability, and unwillingness to involve "outsiders." Because of social isolation, these elderly are also at risk for abuse at the hands of non caregivers. This abuse often takes the form of financial exploitation and extortion.

Elders who live at home alone are at risk for self-abuse or neglect or abuse and neglect by a continuing-care health provider. The theoretical models are of only limited utility in these cases. These elders may well be very dependent and have a number of impairments that lead to inadequate care, and therefore, the impairment theories may help identify elders who are high risk. This inadequate care, however, may evolve from the elder's inability to take care of his or her own daily needs. Another potential source of inadequate care may be a primary physician who is not monitoring the elder's needs adequately or a visiting nurse service that is not maintaining the care needed. If there are neighbors involved who are providing a caregiver role, the elder becomes a part of the second category (at home with others). The theoretical models of stressed caretaker, psychopathology of the abuser, and transgenerational violence do not fit for the elder at home alone. We do know that an elder living at home alone can get into great difficulty, particularly in the realm of self-neglect. This situation is often insidious, and over a period of time the elder's functional capabilities and health status can decline to a degree that the elder can no longer maintain his or her own health and well being. The most difficult aspect of this situation is the access issue, which has already been discussed.

There are several potentially effective intervention strategies for prevention of inadequate care which need to be explored. Some relate to changes in the existing social and medical service systems so that fewer barriers are created for the elderly person to overcome in order to access services. Transportation services, availability of same day scheduling for multiple specialty visits, provision of in home services, use of an ombudsmen to help elderly persons navigate the maze of social and medical services would help to lower barriers to care. Aggressive outreach by governmental programs to identify elderly clients who are eligible for services but not receiving them. This suggestion is not popular with those who seek to reduce government expenditures by restricting access. The creation of new housing which facilitates the clustering of services and less isolation is also likely to be effective.

Other strategies derive from exchange theory and apply to abuse. Interventions which reduce social isolation will probably be effective in preventing abuse. Innovative surveillance programs such as the U.S. Postal Service monitoring system are good examples. Each day as the postman delivers mail, he or she checks to be sure that the elderly person is all right, and if not, gets the individual help in a timely fashion. Another program that could benefit elders could be modeled on lifeline, the telephone network service that enables the elderly person to notify medical or protective service assistance. Other programs operating on the block or neighborhood level supported by local agencies on aging need to be developed to help reduce social isolation.

Exchange theory also predicts that if the penalties for abuse are increased then its frequency will decrease. Effective prevention might be enhanced by changes in the criminal statutes regarding extortion, theft, and battering involving elderly victims. By increasing penalties and raising the priority assigned to these cases by the police and prosecuters, a more effective deterrent might be established.

ELDERS AT HOME WITH OTHERS

Elderly people who live at home with others fall into two subcategories: (a) Those who live at home with caregivers such as spouses, offspring, grandchildren, friends, or paid care-providers, and (b) those who live at home with others who do not provide a caregiver role.

In the first group, the caregivers have a responsibility, whether formal or informal, to that elder and provide services to the elder. In this group each of the theoretical models can apply. If inadequate care results due to dependencies of the elder or due to a stressed caretaker situation, the first intervention that should be employed is provision of support services for the caretaker as well as the elder. These services may take the form of respite care, elder day-care, domestic services, or other social services that lighten the perceived burden of the caregiver. If the inadequate care results from psychopathology of the abuser, interventions will need to be directed toward resolving the pathology or removing the abuser from the elder's residence. Obviously, the other option is to remove the elder. However, we would like to suggest that this practice is all too common and should be viewed as a last resort unless it is specifically requested by the elder. Inadequate care due to a transgenerational violence pattern will need intervention based on the nature of the event. Assault and battery is against the law and criminal proceedings may need to be instituted in such cases. Less black and white situations may need a careful evaluation by clinicians or protective service workers in order to sort out the appropriate intervention. If social isolation is the issue for elders at home with caregivers, casefinding and access issues will take priority. Whenever possible, the approach should be nonjudgmental with a keen sense of awareness for the elder's preferences in relation to resolving the inadequate care issues.

Group B elders include those such as the aging grandmother who is in relatively good health and allows her children or grandchildren to live with her for the purpose of providing them with a place to live. One issue for this group is whether or not a caregiving relationship can be established between the elder and the other person or persons living with that elder. In the event that the elder is living at home with noncaregivers, intervention strategies will depend on the individual situation. If the elder is competent and voices concern about actions of the noncaregiver living in the household, it will be important to encourage the elder to think through whether or not he or she would like to have the other individual removed from the home. An example of this might be a grandparent who allows a grandson or granddaughter to live with him or her without the exchange of any services. While the elder is likely to benefit from this informal surveillance mechanism, he or she may also be at risk for extortion, robbery, assault, or battery. The theories that would apply in this situation are debatable. The impairment theories and stressed caretaker theory would not apply as there is no exchange of services in this scenario. The psychopathology of the abuser theory as well as the transgenerational violence theory could apply. Removal of the noncaregiver through the legal system or removal of the elder from the situation may be necessary. The latter example might occur if the elder willingly decided to sell his or her home and move into a smaller apartment, for example. Extreme sensitivity would be necessary in this case to be certain that the elder felt he or she had a choice and were in control of the decision making. The social isolation theory could apply to the elder at home with a noncaregiver in the same way as it applies to elders at home with caregivers.

Clinicians have found empirically that bringing outside help into the home reduces abuse and neglect independently of any contribution these services might make to meeting the elderly person's care needs. This suggests that by reducing social isolation and by increasing the likelihood of reporting abuse or neglect abuse can be ameliorated. It is likely that the same strategy can be used to prevent abuse if such services can be put into place prospectively. In order to do this, we need to develop more accurate profiles of the high risk elder so that interventions can be targeted.

In addition to the strategies discussed in the first section, another avenue of approach is to reduce the dependency of the abusing caretaker on the elderly person for financial support, a common situation. A serious attempt to prevent abuse and neglect will require the development of mechanisms to provide financial support for families to permit them to care for their elderly parents. Many other countries pay families for homecare services they provide to their elderly relatives. Families often have to give up employment or otherwise forfeit income in order to provide care. It is important that the caretaking role of the family be supported. The corollary is that the need to misappropriate the elderly person's resources would also be lessened thereby reducing the 'benefit' derived from abuse.

INSTITUTIONAL SETTINGS

Elders who live in institutional settings may also be at risk for inadequate care. While exposés of nursing homes have provided sensational accounts of elder abuse in those settings, such events are not the norm and are often blown out of proportion by the media. Unfortunately, however, inadequate care can occur in institutional settings such as rest homes, nursing homes, and hospitals, and needs to be considered a possibility.

Rest homes are a special situation. They are a quasi-

institutional setting in that they are licensed by departments of public health. However, there is' no requirement
that a health care professional be on the premises. In fact,
elders who reside in a rest home are supposed to be able to
perform all their activities of daily living independently. The
licensing requirements vary from state to state, but the
important aspect in this living situation is that there is no
contract for health care services of a skilled nature. In this
setting each of the theoretical models of inadequate care can
apply. Impairment theories and stressed caretaker theories
can apply in that the responsible person (R.P.) in the rest
home may become overwhelmed by growing demands from
elders who are declining in health. Acts of abuse or neglect
may occur. The psychopathology of the abuser theory and
the transgenerational violence theory may also apply in this
situation if the responsible person is being abusive. The
abuse may take any number of forms ranging from assault
to extortion and such facilities need to be monitored on a
regular basis. State agencies need to proactively identify
rest homes that are incapable of meeting the demands posed
by the elders living there. The social isolation theory may
also hold in this setting. Even though rest homes provide
group living, a situation could evolve where the responsible
person intimidates the elders as a group, and there can
evolve a "conspiracy of silence" where the elders fear retri-
bution. As a group they may remain silent about the actions
of the responsible person at the rest home. State agencies
responsible for licensing rest homes need to alert their staff
to the possibility of such a situation so that appropriate
surveillance activities can ensue. A resident's bill of rights
similar to a patient's bill of rights can be useful for the
purpose of alerting rest home residents to their rights.

Nursing homes and hospitals differ from rest homes in
that there is a contract between the elder and the institution
that good care will be provided. While the social isolation
theory does not hold in these institutions, each of the other
theoretical models may apply as reasons for inadequate care
in such institutions. In nursing homes, it is well known that

elders are more frail, debilitated, and dependent. The turn-over rate for employees in such institutions is frequently very rapid and there has been documentation of job dissat-isfaction in these settings. Some would argue that the social isolation theory does apply in that if an elderly resident has frequent visitors, he or she is less isolated and better cared for. A case could be made for this if social isolation is meant in the context that the elder is otherwise isolated from the outside world. The view stated here looks at the elder as not isolated from other human beings. The impairment theory and stressed caretaker theory are both potential reasons for inadequate care occurring in long-term care. With this in mind, prevention strategies include better staff-to-patient ratios; better salaries for nursing assistants, nurses, and physicians who choose to work in long-term care; and sup-port groups within the work environment that enable health care providers to discuss their feelings about stress-ful situations. These opportunities for discussion should be conducted in a relaxed, nonthreatening environment where care providers truly feel supported and do not fear that their jobs will be in jeopardy if they admit that there are days when delivering care to multiply impaired elders is difficult. Short leaves of absence should be allowed when health care workers in long-term care feel that they need a break and yet may not have accrued the necessary vacation days to get the rest they may need so desperately in order to approach their job with renewed energy. Care providers in long-term care should also have the opportunity to say honestly when they have a personality conflict with particu-lar elders and feel that they are unable to give good care if they do not get along. This choice is usually not an option and may contribute to inadequate care in that neglect may ensue.

The psychopathology of the abuser and transgenerational violence theories of inadequate care may apply as well. If a care provider is found to be a known drug abuser, alcoholic, or have a significant mental illness that impairs his or her ability to give good care, he or she needs to be removed from the workplace. Remedial interventions should be offered to the care provider, but the first issue at hand is the safety and well being of the elder.

Reducing social isolation and increasing the penalties for providing inadequate care are the most common approaches used to prevent abuse and neglect in nursing homes and other long term care institutions. Similar constraints and programs usually do not include unlicensed facilities such as rest homes. Given the prevalence of abuse and neglect in other settings, it will be important to obtain data regarding the incidence of abuse in rest homes and make the necessary changes in state licensing laws if the incidence is significant. Developing national standards that could be applied to nursing home care would be a helpful step in reducing institutional abuse and neglect by providing a clear expectation of what constitutes adequate care. Sanctions already exist that make abuse and neglect extremely costly to institutions. The issue is to identify potential cases and homes with substandard care before serious harm is done.

SUMMARY

Ultimately the prevention of inadequate care of the elderly is a political issue. Many of the most effective strategies will require a reallocation of society's resource. Adequate income support for the elderly so they can purchase services, availability of health care and health care insurance, and financial support for family caretakers all require money. Without a consensus that abuse, neglect, and inadequate care of the elderly are serious problems worthy of attention, resources will not be found. All individuals involved in eliminating inadequate care of the elderly need to pursue political action as well as their professional activities, because ultimately, abuse and neglect will diminish when society places a higher value on the well being of its elderly citizens.

REFERENCES

Branch, L. G. (1980). *Vulnerable Elders*. Gerontological Monograph #6. Washington, DC: Gerontological Society of America.

Gelles, R. J. (1982, February). Applying Research on Family Violence to Clinical Practice. *Journal of Marriage and the Family, 44*(1), 9-20.

Rathbone-McCuan, E. (1980, May). Elderly Victims of Family Violence and Neglect. *Social Casework: The Journal of Contemporary Social Work, 61*(5), 296-304.

Snyder, J. C., Bowles, R. T., & Newberger, E. H. (1982). Improving Research and Practice on Family Violence. *Urban and Social Change Review, 15*(2), 3-7.

U.S. Department of Health and Human Services, Public Health Service. (1984). *Report on Education and Training in Geriatrics and Gerontology.* Administrative document. Bethesda, MD: National Institute on Aging.

U.S. Senate, Special Committee on Aging. (1984). *Aging America: Trends and Projections.* Washington, DC: U.S. Senate, Special Committee on Aging in conjunction with the American Association of Retired Persons.

Appendix A

Development of the Elder Assessment Instrument (EAI)

The development of the Elder Assessment Instrument (EAI) began in August 1981 by Terry T. Fulmer. At that time, the first Massachusetts reporting law was enacted (Chapter 479 of the General Laws) which mandated reporting of any suspected cases of elder abuse, neglect, or mistreatment of elders in long-term-care settings. Prompted by this law, the EAI project was undertaken for the purpose of constructing a reliable and valid tool for assessing these cases. It should be noted here that the EAI went through several revision processes before taking the form presented in Chapter 3 of this book.

PHASE 1

During August 1981, a one-month pilot project was conducted in the emergency unit at Boston's Beth Israel Hospital, in order to test the initial assessment instrument, detect any cases of suspected elder abuse, and examine any training deficits in staff nurses participating in the study. Staff training was necessary before the pilot project began, in order to ensure the nurses had a common understanding of elder abuse and were familiar with the cardinal signs and symptoms of abuse. An in-service program was given by known experts in the field of elder abuse. In addition, each emergency unit nurse was given a training packet that included a copy of the Massachusetts reporting law, journal articles on the subject, and a copy of the pilot assessment instrument with specific instructions for screening. Staff meetings were held prior to the proposed one-month pilot project, in order to clarify any misconceptions and answer any questions.

The pilot screening instrument (which preceded the Elder Assessment Instrument reproduced in Chapter 3—Chapter 3 describing a later and more refined version) was incorporated into the assessment of all emergency unit patients over 70 years of age. The instrument was placed in each elder's chart by the registration secretary, and the emergency unit nurse was responsible for completion of the instrument. All suspected cases were referred to the hospital elder abuse team. During that month, 161 elder assessment forms were collected. Thirty-four percent of those forms were completely filled out ($N = 55$), 28 percent were partially completed ($N = 45$), and 38 percent ($N = 61$) were left blank due to a lack of time.

Section I of the instrument contained six questions: 1 through 3 pertained to demographic data, 4 and 6 related to reason for admission, and 5 was an assessment of the patient's mental status. Section II contained assessment questions related to dependency needs, psychological and material aspects of the elder, and caregiver interactions noted. Section III contained physical signs known to be indicators of potential abuse of the elderly, and Section IV contained questions regarding medications and their administration. Section V asked the nurse to make a general assessment as to whether, in his or her opinion, the patient had been abused, neglected, or mistreated prior to admission to the Beth Israel Hospital. Finally, Sections VI and VII provided for summary and outcome statements.

At the end of the month the nursing staff provided feedback regarding the utility of the instrument and gave suggestions for revision. They reported that the instrument was useful but could be utilized better in a checklist format with less narrative. Questions that were unclear, poorly worded, or redundant were corrected, and a checklist assessment instrument was constructed.

PHASE 2

A second pilot study utilizing the same age guidelines and process was conducted between April 1982 and August 1982, using the revised instrument. There were 484 individuals who were screened for elder abuse, neglect, or mistreatment. The second pilot instrument asked the nurse to rate the assessment variables (previously described) as "good," "fair," or "poor." Since these categories enabled the researcher to measure the results on an ordinal scale only, it was not possible to perform any meaningful data analysis in terms of significant differences among patients. However, these data were reported in terms of trends noted, and a content validity index (CVI) of 0.83 was determined, utilizing Waltz and Bausell's CVI index (1981).

The CVI index required two or more independent professionals to rate the relevance of each item on the EAI on a four-point scale ranging from "not relevant" to "very relevant." The CVI was then defined as the proportion of items given a rating of "quite relevant" or "very relevant" by the raters. The CVI rating scale for this instrument was given to 12 independent raters who were known to be knowledgeable in the area of elder abuse. The raters came from Beth Israel as well as the Massachusetts General Hospital and the Brigham and Women's Hospital in Boston. This diversity of agencies was felt to be important in order to control for agency bias. In addition, the mix of professionals utilized included five nurses, four physicians, and three social workers, which provided an interdisciplinary point of view.

The content validity score was strong and supported the items in the Elder Assessment Instrument, and therefore, it was appropriate to continue to the next phase.

PHASE 3

The third phase of the EAI construction concerned revamping the instrument format in order to obtain meaningful statistical analyses and an inter-rater reliability (IRR) index. This was completed during February 1983, with the items of the previous EAI organized into a more sensitive rating scale. The demographic variables were retained in their former presentation, but the items listed under each of the nine general sections of the instrument required ratings on a five-point Likert scale ranging from positive to negative. This adjustment yielded a data set that could undergo more sophisticated statistical analysis. This time, an IRR index as outlined by Waltz and Bausell (1981) could be calculated. This index refers to the agreement between the raters in assigning scores to the responses being judged and requires that two independent raters score the responses in question. By calculating the IRR for 20 EAI's from inpatients at the Beth Israel Hospital, a Pearson correlation coefficient of .83 was determined, which indicates a high degree of inter-rater reliability. The 20 IRR assessments were conducted by two independent raters over the course of three days. Prior consent was given by the patients, and this phase was approved by the Committee of Clinical Investigations.

Concurrently, during February 1983, the third revision of the EAI was tested in the emergency unit in the same manner as described previously for the first two versions. A total of 160 elders over 70 years of age were available for assessment that month, with around 146 EAI's completed.

The analysis of the 146 cases from the February 1983 EAI is described in Chapter 3. This group of elders scored more positively on the EAI than the scores from elders referred to the Elder Assessment Team.

These findings enhance the desirability of the EAI's use and provide health care practitioners with an assurance that it is an instrument that demonstrates acceptable psychometric properties. It will be important for other researchers in the field to provide the same kind of analysis of the instruments they choose, in order to promote their utility and applicability.

In summary, the Elder Assessment Instrument is one that has been revised over a period of three years utilizing standard psychometric testing on data from the clinical field. It is hoped that other researchers will retest its utility in their own settings.

Appendix B

Massachusetts Elder Protective Services Program, Assessment and Functional Evaluation Form

PART I: BASIC INFORMATION

Protective Service Agency: _____ Intake Date: _____
Client ID# _____ Date of Initial Visit_____
Caseworker _____ Where? _____

Key Facts:
1. Name _____
2. Address _____
3. Telephone # _____
4. Social Security # _____
5. English Spoken:
   Yes _____ No _____
   Principal Language If Not
   English: _____

6. Sex _____
7. Date of Birth _____
8. Ethnicity (optional) _____
9. Religion (optional) _____
10. Lives with _____
_____
_____
_____

11. *Emergency Contacts:*
   a. Name _____
      Address _____
      Town/City _____
      Relationship _____
      Telephone # _____

   b. Name _____
      Address _____
      Town/City _____
      Relationship _____
      Telephone # _____

12. *Medical Resources*:
    Hospital _____   Telephone # _____
    Primary Doctor _____   Telephone # _____

13. *Other Resources*
    _____   Telephone # _____
    _____   Telephone # _____
    _____   Telephone # _____
    _____   Telephone # _____

14. *Financial Category*:   15. *Health Care Coverage*:
    ☐ Income Eligible   ☐ Medicare # _____
    ☐ SSI/OAA, DA, AB   1-Part A 2-Part B
      (circle one)   Medicaid # _____
    ☐ Sliding Fee: Amount _____   ☐ Medex 1 2 3 # _____
      Annual Income _____   ☐ Other _____

16. *Alleged Perpetrator*:   17. *Alleged Perpetrator*:
    Name _____   _____
    Address _____   _____
    Relation _____   _____
    Telephone # _____   _____

PART II: ASSESSMENT OF SERIOUS PHYSICAL OR EMOTIONAL ABUSE AND NEGLECT

PRES-Present
PROB-Probable
UNK-Unknown
ABS-Absent

	PRES	PROB	UNK	ABS	NARRATIVE (Note source and date)
A. Evidence of Serious Physical Abuse					
1. Bruises, Welts	3	2	1	0	_____
2. Sprains, Dislocations	3	2	1	0	
3. Burns, Scalding	3	2	1	0	_____
4. Abrasions, Lacerations	3	2	1	0	
5. Wounds, Cuts, Punctures	3	2	1	0	_____

	P	P				
	R	R	U	A		
A. Evidence of Serious	E	O	N	B	NARRATIVE	
Physical Abuse	S	B	K	S	(Note source and date)	

	PRES	PROB	UNK	ABS	
6. Broken Bones	3	2	1	0	_____
7. Internal Injuries	3	2	1	0	_____
8. Sexual Assault	3	2	1	0	_____
9. Other	3	2	1	0	_____

_____

_____

_____

_____

_____

_____

_____

B. Evidence of Serious Emotional Abuse	PRES	PROB	UNK	ABS	NARRATIVE (Note source and date)
1. Sleep Disturbance	3	2	1	0	
2. Worried, Anxious	3	2	1	0	_____
3. Irritable, Easily Upset	3	2	1	0	
4. Change in Eating Habits	3	2	1	0	_____
5. Loss of Interest	3	2	1	0	
6. Fear of Retribution	3	2	1	0	_____
7. Suicidal Talk, Wishes	3	2	1	0	
8. Shaking, Trembling and/or Crying Frequently	3	2	1	0	_____
9. Other	3	2	1	0	_____

_____

_____

_____

_____

_____

C. Abusive Actions (Emotional and Physical)					NARRATIVE (Note source and date)
1. Insulted, swore, or yelled at victim	3	2	1	0	_____
2. Threatened, Coerced	3	2	1	0	_____
3. Confined/Isolated	3	2	1	0	
4. Attempted to harm	3	2	1	0	_____
5. Threw Objects at Victim	3	2	1	0	
6. Pushed, Grabbed Victim	3	2	1	0	_____
7. Struck or Kicked Victim	3	2	1	0	
8. Threatened Victim with Weapon	3	2	1	0	_____
9. Injured Victim with Weapon	3	2	1	0	_____
10. Other	3	2	1	0	_____

_____

_____

_____

_____

_____

_____

	P R E S	P R O B	R U N K	A B S	NARRATIVE (Note source and date)
D. Evidence of Serious Neglect					
1. Dirt, Fleas, or Lice on Person	3	2	1	0	
2. Skin Rashes	3	2	1	0	_____
3. Sores	3	2	1	0	
4. Malnourished	3	2	1	0	_____
5. Dehydrated	3	2	1	0	
6. Inappropriate Clothing	3	2	1	0	_____
7. Fecal/Urine Smell	3	2	1	0	
8. Untreated Medical Condition	3	2	1	0	_____
9. Other	3	2	1	0	

E. Neglectful Actions

Failure to Provide: _____

	PRES	PROB	RUNK	ABS	
1. Adequate Food	3	2	1	0	
2. Adequate Heat	3	2	1	0	_____
3. Adequate Personal Care	3	2	1	0	
4. Adequate Supervision	3	2	1	0	_____
5. a. Prescribed Medication	3	2	1	0	
b. Medical Equipment or Aids	3	2	1	0	_____
c. Other Medical Services	3	2	1	0	
6. Other	3	2	1	0	_____

F. Financial Exploitation	P R E S	P R O B	U N K	A B S	NARRATIVE (Note source and date)
1. Mismanagement of Victim's Income	3	2	1	0	
2. Misappropriation of Victim's Income	3	2	1	0	_____
3. Other	3	2	1	0	_____

G. Physical Environment Problems

	P R E S	P R O B	U N K	A B S	
1. Repair	3	2	1	0	_____
2. Level of Cleanliness	3	2	1	0	
3. Architectural Barriers	3	2	1	0	
4. Kitchen/Bathroom Facilities	3	2	1	0	
5. Living/Sleeping Area	3	2	1	0	_____
6. Utilities	3	2	1	0	
7. Fire Safety	3	2	1	0	_____
8. Pest Control	3	2	1	0	
9. Other	3	2	1	0	_____

PART III: FUNCTIONAL EVALUATION

A. Current Medical Conditions: ( ) if Diagnosed

1. ( ) _____
2. ( ) _____
3. ( ) _____
4. ( ) _____
5. ( ) _____

B. Recent Hospitalizations: *Dates:*

1. _____   _____
2. _____   _____
3. _____   _____
4. _____   _____

C. Current Medical Treatment/Therapies (by self or others):

1. _____
2. _____
3. _____
4. _____

D. Current Medications:

	Date	Name	Dosage/Frequency	Purpose	Doctor	Pharmacy
1.						
2.						
3.						
4.						
5.						
6.						

E. Activities of Daily Living

( ) Home Care Intervention	How Does Client Usually: (Circle One)
☐	1. *Bathe* 0 Completely able 1 Able with aids/difficulty 2 Able with helper 3 Unable
☐	2. *Dress/Undress* 0 Completely able 1 Able with aids/difficulty 2 Able with helper 3 Unable

F. Instrumental Activities of Daily Living

( ) Home Care Intervention	Describe What Client Can Do (Circle One)
☐	1. *Meal Preparation* 0 Without help 1 With some help 2 Can't do at all
☐	2. *Housework* 0 Without help 1 With some help 2 Can't do at all
☐	3. *Laundry* 0 Without help 1 With some help 2 Can't do at all
☐	4. *Shopping* 0 Without help 1 With some help 2 Can't do at all

E. Activities of Daily Living

( ) Home Care Intervention	How Does Client Usually: (Circle One)
☐	3. *Eat* 0 Completely able 1 Able with aids/difficulty 2 Able with helper 3 Unable
☐	4. *Toilet* 0 Completely able 1 Able with aids/difficulty 2 Able with helper 3 Unable
☐	5. *Continence*

	Bladder	Bowel
	0 Complete control	0
	1 Self-care devices, no accidents	1
	2 Helper, occasional accidents	2
	3 Incontinent	3

F. Instrumental Activities of Daily Living

( ) Home Care Intervention	Describe What Client Can Do (Circle One)
☐	5. *Taking Medicine* 0 Without help 1 With some help 2 Can't do at all
☐	6. *Get Around Outside* 0 Without help 1 With some help 2 Can't do at all
☐	7. *Transportation* 0 Without help 1 With some help 2 Can't do at all
☐	8. *Money Management* 0 Without help 1 With some help 2 Can't do at all
☐	9. *Use Telephone* 0 Without help 1 With some help 2 Can't do at all

( ) Home Care Intervention	How Does Client Usually: (Circle One)	( ) Home Care Intervention	Describe What Client Can Do (Circle One)
☐	6. *Transfer In/Out/ Bed/Chair* 0 Completely able 1 Able with aids/diffi-culty 2 Able with helper 3 Unable		
☐	7. *Get Around Inside* 0 Completely able 1 Able with aids/diffi-culty 2 Able with helper 3 Unable		

Y- Yes
S- Sometimes   NARRATIVE
N-No   (Note source and date)

G. Cognitive Functioning   Y   S   N
   1. Oriented to time   3   2   1
   2. Oriented to place   3   2   1
   3. Oriented to people   3   2   1
   4. Recent memory loss   3   2   1
   5. Distant memory loss   3   2   1
   6. Inappropriate judg-   3   2   1
     ments
   7. Able to communicate   3   2   1
   8. Able to comprehend   3   2   1

H. Psychiatric History
   1. *Hospitalizations:*   *Date:*
     a. _____   / /
     b. _____   / /
     c. _____   / /
   2. *Recent/Current Treatment*
     Provider(s):   *Date:*
     a. _____   / /
     b. _____   / /
     c. _____   / /

                  Y   N   UNK
I. Capacity to Consent   3   2   1

J. Capacity Assessed By: *Date:*
   1. _____   / /
   2. _____   / /

K. Fiduciary Relationships:
   (*Guard, Cons., Prot., Power Atty., Payee*)
               Court   Date(s)
   1. _____
   2. _____

PART IV: RISK FACTORS
PRES-Present
PROB-Probable
UNK-Unknown
ABS-Absent

	VICTIM				ABUSER			
	PRES	PROB	UNK	ABS	PRES	PROB	UNK	ABS
1. Live together	3	2	1	0	3	2	1	0
2. Socially isolated	3	2	1	0	3	2	1	0
3. Unable to care for self if left alone	3	2	1	0	3	2	1	0
4. Unable to summon assistance	3	2	1	0	3	2	1	0
5. Unable to ward off attack	3	2	1	0	3	2	1	0
6. Alcohol abuser	3	2	1	0	3	2	1	0
7. Drug abuser	3	2	1	0	3	2	1	0
8. Emotional Problems	3	2	1	0	3	2	1	0
9. Behavioral Problems	3	2	1	0	3	2	1	0
10. Previous Psychiatric Hospitalization	3	2	1	0	3	2	1	0
11. Mentally Retarded	3	2	1	0	3	2	1	0
12. Confused/Disoriented	3	2	1	0	3	2	1	0
13. History of Assaults on Others	3	2	1	0	3	2	1	0
14. Unemployed	3	2	1	0	3	2	1	0
15. Dependency								
a. Personal Care	3	2	1	0	3	2	1	0
b. Income	3	2	1	0	3	2	1	0
c. Financial Management	3	2	1	0	3	2	1	0
d. Emotional	3	2	1	0	3	2	1	0
e. Household Maintenance (cooking, cleaning, etc.)	3	2	1	0	3	2	1	0
f. Transportation	3	2	1	0	3	2	1	0

NARRATIVE
(Note source and date)

_____

_____

_____

_____

_____

_____

_____

_____

_____

_____

_____

_____

_____

_____

_____

_____

_____

_____

_____

_____

_____

PART V: ASSESSMENT OF NEED FOR PROTECTIVE INTERVENTION

1. *Summary of Assessment*

_____
_____
_____
_____
_____
_____

2. *Statement of Reasonable Cause*

_____
_____
_____
_____
_____
_____

PART VI: ACTION TAKEN

A. Case Opened _____   Case Not Opened _____
B. Case Referred to:
   1. Home Care   1 _____ Yes   2 _____ No
   2. Other   1 _____ Yes   2 _____ No
C. Name of Agency _____ Date _____
   Name of Agency _____ Date _____
   Name of Agency _____ Date _____
D. Case Reported to District Attorney   1 _____ Yes   2 _____ No

PART VII: SIGNATURES

Protective Service Worker _____ Date _____
Supervisor _____ Date _____

Index